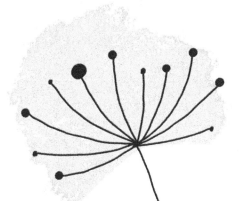

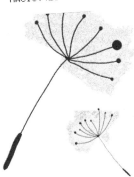

For
Like
Minds

Mental Illness
Recovery
Insights

KATHERINE PONTE

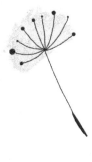

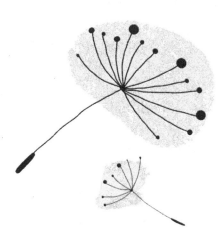

Foreword by
Larry Davidson, Ph.D.
Professor of Psychiatry
School of Medicine
Yale University

Print ISBN: 978-0-578-73161-2

E-ISBN: 978-0-578-73160-5

LCCN: 2020914113

For Like Minds: Mental Illness Recovery Insights includes information that may benefit mental health, but this information is not a substitute for medical advice, diagnosis or treatment provided by a qualified healthcare provider. Always seek the advice of a qualified healthcare provider.

If you or someone you know is experiencing suicidal thoughts, please call the National Suicide Prevention Lifeline at 800-273-8255.

Published in the United States by Real MH Works, LLC

A portion of book sales will be donated to the National Alliance on Mental Illness-New York City.

Table of Contents

Acknowledgments ix

Foreword.. xv

Part I. Our Journey 1

  1 Stigma, Meet Hope 3

  2 Me – and My Wife's Bipolar Diagnosis.. 7

Part II. Self-recognition.. 9

  3 Hope and Recovery 11

  4 Power to Create Change Comes from Within 15

  5 Two Antidotes to Stigma 17

  6 Embracing the Diversity within Us 20

  7 The Stages of My Mental Illness...23

  8 Addressing Emotions with Mental Illness 26

  9 Talking about Mental Illness: Reaching In...................................30

  10 Coming Out about Your Bipolar Disorder 35

  11 The Example Celebrities with Mental Illness Set........................40

Part III. Treatment and Recovery.................................. 43

  12 Finding the Best Psychiatrist for You..45

  13 Hope Starts with Mutual Peer Support 49

  14 The Effectiveness of Peer Support within the Context of Mental Illness 52

  15 Family-to-Family Peer Support 57

  16 Shared Decision-making: Getting a Say in Your Care 62

  17 Families Can Work Together 65

  18 Finding the Best Medication Regimen 69

  19 A Risk Too Big Not to Take: A Story of Recovery.......................73

  20 What Is Recovery? 77

  21 Psychiatric Rehabilitation...82

  22 People with Mental Illness Can Work 88

  23 The Mental Health Movement in the Workplace 92

  24 Mental Health Peer Specialist Support 97

  25 Building Mental Health Resilience..102

  26 Ways to Manage and Cope with Stress 106

27 The Remarkable Human Animal Bond 110

28 Coping with Mental Illness: What Not To Do 115

29 Working on Recovery with Loved Ones 118

30 Learning to Take Care of Myself 121

Part IV. Specific Experiences 125

31 Learning from Past Manias and Avoiding Future Relapses 127

32 Turning Suicidal Ideation into Hope 131

33 Suicide: Saving Lives Now and Beyond 135

34 My Reality During a Psychotic Episode 139

35 Preventing and Preparing for a Mental Health Crisis 143

36 That Time in the Psych Ward 147

Part V. Specific Communities 151

37 Suicide Prevention for College Students 153

38 Parents and their College Child's Mental Health 157

39 Taking a College Medical Leave 161

40 Mental Health Challenges in the LGBTQ+ Community 169

41 Mental Health Challenges in Immigrant Communities 173

Part VI. Rights and Advocacy 177

42 The Many Forms of Mental Illness Discrimination 179

43 Ways We Can Address the Social Determinants of Mental Health 183

44 Mental Health Law Considerations, New York Example 188

45 A Primer on Government Benefits 191

Appendix I. Additional Resources 197

1 Collaborative Care Plan 199

2 The Transtheoretical Model (Stages of Change) 229

3 Active Listening 232

4 Reframing 237

5 SMART Goals 239

6 Mental Health Education 242

7 Mental Health Non-profits 245

8 Suicide Prevention Resources 248

9 Peer Supporters/Peer Specialists 249

10 Additional References in Chapters 253

Appendix II. ForLikeMinds 267

1 ForLikeMinds Explained...269

2 Video Script: A Recovery Journey 274

3 Video Script: Talking About Mental Illness.....................................277

4 Video Script: A Caregiver's Mental Illness Journey 279

5 Bipolar Thriving Bipolar Recovery Coaching..................................285

6 Psych Ward Greeting Cards 288

To Izzy

Acknowledgments

This book is a reflection on my experiences living with severe bipolar I disorder with psychosis for 20 years. I have collected my essays and contributions from esteemed collaborators to turn the struggles I experienced with mental illness into lessons and tools for my peers and their loved ones. It is a form of reconciliation that testifies to my recovery. It also reflects and acknowledges the acts of many who stood by me, lifted me up, and gave me the support and help to reach recovery. I offer these stories as an example that others should find hope in to pursue their own recovery.

My mental illness journey started in 2000 when I was first diagnosed with bipolar. I was in the midst of a severe manic episode while a graduate student at the Wharton School of the University of Pennsylvania. I realized now that a confluence of stressors, including family illness, career uncertainties, academic stress, and a sexual assault likely triggered the episode. But the shock and stigma wouldn't allow me to accept the diagnosis back then.

Left unaddressed, my emotional health chipped at my academic performance. I lost self-esteem and self-worth. I isolated myself. Eventually, I was left with one friend, but he was lifesaving - Nuno Pereira. Nuno would not allow me to fade into the shadows of my depression. He drew me out of hiding. He forced me to engage. He was always there to listen and support me. His nudges and help kept me in the game. I also had Professor Paul Kleindorfer who was as brilliant as he was kind. He put things in perspective for me. He emphasized that my today would not be my forever, and that many more important days lay beyond. Jane Thompson, who worked in the Vice Dean's office, knew of my challenges from her role but went beyond it with her care and comfort. She helped and supported me when I was at my worst – taking me to lunch for my birthday when I was in the depths of my depression. I remember her running on the convocation field to hug me at graduation.

After graduating, I returned home to New York City. Over the next six years, I continued to refuse all treatment. I lived in deep depression. I had extended periods of suicidal ideation. Fortunately, I had the constant companionship of my beloved cat, Dude. His affection, unflinching devotion, and love helped me through my darkest moments. I couldn't bear the thought of being without my family or him, so I lived on.

And eventually – weeks, months, or years later – I would cycle up, the other part of bipolar. Over the years, there were several furious manic episodes leading to three involuntary hospitalizations. My psychosis during one of these episodes led to my arrest. And once the storm inside me passed, I was left to pick up the pieces and rebuild slowly once again.

Through it all, the love and support of my spouse Izzy never wavered. He's been by my side through the saddest and happiest times of my life. He is an important part of all I do. He has given voice to caregivers not only to recognize their contributions but also to promote peer support among them. His empathy and compassion for our mental illness community – those with conditions and their supporters – is boundless. He is a great inspiration to me.

My parents were always there for me too. Their faith was a constant presence and force in my journey. They kept faith that my mental illness had not taken away the person I always was, and it lifted me up. They shared the light from their hope when mine was extinguished. They showed me the tremendous power that family love can have in the lives of those with mental illness. I would have never survived those hardest years without Izzy, my parents and my Dude. I am here, because of all of them.

My last hospitalization led to an awakening – to the possibility of recovery. Throughout my first 14 years of living with mental illness, I had never seen an example of someone living with serious mental illness in recovery. Chaya Weinstein, an occupational therapist at the Payne Whitney Clinic, New York-Presbyterian Hospital in New York City showed me that example during my last hospitalization. She showed me the value of peer support. She sparked that tiny flicker of hope within me. There should be a Chaya in every psychiatric unit. Her love and commitment to her patients is inspiring. And now that I am in recovery, we collaborate on projects. She saw me as a person, not just a patient in the psych ward or my illness.

Following my last discharge, my hope grew strong enough for me to see that I had to live a full and meaningful life. It became clear to me that there was one remaining obstacle to my getting well - my highly esteemed psychiatrist. I realized that her treatment approach had been discouraging, stigmatizing and deferring my recovery. After many years of treatment, I finally terminated our relationship.

I obsessively and desperately searched for a psychiatrist who could treat me to live my best life. I was blessed to find a caring and loving doctor in Dr. Joseph Goldberg. He too treated me as a person and not a diagnosis. He allowed me to define my goals and treated me to achieve those goals. Within six months, I was truly on my way – a medication regimen that finally worked, a more active lifestyle, better relationships with my friends and family, and the confidence to pursue an ambitious career. He gave me my life back.

Through these struggles, I didn't have many friends, but two that stuck with me, Rui Pires and Fabíola Costa Girão, more than made up for those I lost. They were with me throughout my struggles and achievements. They were always there for me – to talk, listen, and sit with me. They always had time for me even when the talk was sad and somber. They forced me to see when things were not as bad as I lamented. They reminded me that I mattered and was cared for. I wish all people with mental illness had friends like Rui and Fabíola.

Once I realized that my recovery was not fleeting, with Izzy's invaluable help, I built an online peer support community, ForLikeMinds. I wanted to make it easier for others to access the peer support that became so critical to my own recovery. I built it, and people came, people living with mental illness and their supporters. Having supporters be part of my mission was always extremely important to me. I also created a bipolar recovery coaching service called Bipolar Thriving to help families who are going through the same experiences that my spouse and I did. I want them to avoid some of the mistakes we made and reach recovery more quickly and easily.

As my health improved, I wanted to rejoin the community and engage in the public service that had been so meaningful to me before I became sick. I was ecstatic to join the National Alliance on Mental Illness family. I joined the NAMI-NYC Board who warmly welcomed me, especially the board president Nathan Romano, and shared their own family experiences with mental illness. Nathan encouraged and helped me recognize my potential to address stigma and advocate for better mental health policy at an institutional level. The board appreciates and respects my insights as someone living with mental illness. I am also especially thankful to the support of Matt Kudish, NAMI-NYC's executive director. He has encouraged me in all of my endeavors and helped me overcome my self-doubts. Wanting to share my lessons with a broader audience, I turned to my love of research and writing. I am so grateful to Luna Greenstein, my wonderful editor at the NAMI blog for allowing me to share my story and for amplifying my voice. She's always allowed me to write about what I feel is important and strongly supported my work. Her great insights and editorial skills have helped bring my writing to a broader audience maximizing its impact. Richele Keas, also with NAMI, has been a great source of encouragement for which I am also very grateful. I am truly blessed to be a part of the NAMI family.

I also wanted to show that recovery is possible based on academic rigor and evidentiary support, not just my personal experience. So I turned to the work of Professor Larry Davidson, Professor of Psychiatry, School of Medicine, Yale University, the leading mental health recovery scholar. His work over 30 years has helped many people living with mental illness live better lives. I wish there were more scholars like him with a deep heartfelt commitment to our community. I am extremely grateful for all of the encouragement and support he's provided for me to better understand peer support and recovery and its benefits.

I have also built on the work of ForLikeMinds to share my example and lessons with others in like circumstances. I visit patients in psychiatric units in New York City to share my recovery story of hope and distribute donated greeting cards to the patients. I have personally met with and spoken to over 500 patients. It's my favorite initiative. These patients have truly been one of my greatest sources of inspiration. I am honored by the time I am allowed to spend with them. They remind me of the courage and strength, the hope that burns deep within all people living with mental illness - that no matter the depths of one's pain and suffering, recovery is possible. They remind me of my own journey and the journey that is possible and lies ahead for many of them. I am extremely grateful to Chaya Weinstein and Dawn Beverley at the Payne Whitney Clinic, New York-Presbyterian Hospital and Maryanne Dipasquale and Kristin Sharkey at Lenox Hill Hospital for making my visits possible. I am also very grateful for the collaborations with Fountain House and NAMI-NYC on this initiative.

I have been moved and touched by the tremendous recognition I have received on all of my initiatives. Since I launched ForLikeMinds in 2018, nearly every day someone, both people living with mental illness and their loved ones, has reached out to me to tell me I've given them hope. At times, it is difficult to hold back my tears. I want to thank each and every one of these people for also inspiring my work, showing me that my life has meaning and purpose and that my work is helping many.

I have my life back now. I am firmly living in recovery. My mental illness took a lot away from me, but it gave me so much more. It gave me a deeper appreciation for life's meaning. It made realize the deep love that exists among friends and family. I am blessed to have all of these people in my life, especially Izzy and my parents. They have enabled me to have and share an example of life with mental illness that might inspire and inform others like me.

I want all people with mental illness to know that we all have reasons to be proud of ourselves, that we are loved, that we are worthy of living our best lives – worthy of happiness. Please never lose that hope within you, never doubt it. Hope makes the impossible possible.

Katherine Ponte

Foreword

I have been waiting for over 30 years for someone to write a book like this. That is as long as I have been a mental health professional working with persons experiencing serious mental illnesses. During and shortly after my training, I thought that my job was to "treat" the mental illnesses my patients were experiencing and that their role, if they had a role to play at all, was to do what they were told—which in those days was to take their medications as prescribed and to "avoid stress." The so-called Mental Health Consumer/Survivor Movement was at that time just coming in to its own, making the argument that persons with mental illnesses needed to be empowered to take back control of their own lives from paternalistic and coercive systems of mental health care, but the Movement itself offered people little guidance as to how to do that. Meanwhile, I was just beginning to learn from my own patients and from friends in the Movement what it was like to actually live with a mental health condition and the wide range of challenges that came along with the diagnosis. People had to find their own ways to manage distressing symptoms, unstable moods, and only loosely linked ways of thinking about their condition, all the while having to maintain a meaningful life in the face of poverty, stigma and discrimination, prolonged unemployment, unstable or unsafe housing, family rejection, and social isolation. What the mental health system had to offer was of little help with the day-to-day issues people faced, and mental health advocates were mostly angry about how they had been treated by overwhelmed and under-prepared mental health professionals … such as myself.

It's a wonder that anyone got better under these circumstances, but there was a source of hope and inspiration in the fact that many people recover nonetheless. However, this was mostly on their own and despite rather than because of mental health professionals—people who were almost entirely well-meaning, well-intended individuals, but who didn't have a clue as to what it was like to have to deal with a mental health condition and the various other challenges that came along with it described above. It was at that point that it started to dawn on people like me that we could actually learn the most about recovery from the people themselves who were recovering, both recovering from a mental illness and recovering a meaningful life in their communities. Katherine Ponte is one such person, and she, like many others, had at first to figure out a lot of this wisdom on her own, with minimal assistance or support from mental health professionals like me.

What is different about Katherine, and a small group of like-minded others with similar experiences, is that she then did two very uncommon things. One, she used her accumulating knowledge of what works for her to educate interested and appropriately humble mental health professionals as to how they could be more useful to the people they serve. And two, she turned around and decided to offer her still-accumulating wisdom about self-care to people in similar circumstances and their loved ones. In ways I have seldom seen before, she has taken her hard-won accomplishments in learning how to manage a potentially disabling mental illness in the process of living a whole and gratifying life and offered them in bite size and easily accessible pieces to the people most in need of both inspiration and role modeling. She has truly "been there" in these other people's shoes and is generous in offering them a hand and leading them step by step through many of the lessons she has had to learn mostly on her own. Following her lead, her husband Izzy similarly offers guidance and suggestions to the most important figures in such people's lives, their family and loved ones. What results is an instructive and very practical guide to overcoming the day-to-day challenges of persons living with mental health conditions, from finding the best psychiatrist and medication regimen to finding ways to cope and not to cope with stress and mental illnesses to learning how to take care of oneself, including how to prevent and prepare for future mental health crises.

This is a book I wish I could have had 30 years ago, which distills lessons learned from creative, dogged, and prolonged efforts to find a way to build and maintain a full life in the face of a serious illness. I would suggest that these efforts were almost heroic in nature, except for the fact that Katherine's stories and lessons learned are at their core fundamental to what makes a person fully human. This book is filled with everyday practical wisdom which is directly applicable to the everyday lives of persons living with mental illnesses and their loved ones. It does not require superhuman intelligence or Herculean efforts to put these lessons into action. In retrospect, they may even seem to be nothing but "common sense." But given the sad history of mental health services and the potentially tragic nature of serious mental illnesses, Katherine and her accrued practical wisdom are anything but common.

Give the lessons and guidance offered in this rich and easily accessible book a chance to improve and enhance your life, or the life of a loved one, and you will not regret it. In fact, you too might wish that you had come across such a book much earlier in your own struggles.

Larry Davidson, Ph.D., New Haven, Connecticut

Larry Davidson, Ph.D. is a Professor of Psychiatry and Director of the Program for Recovery and Community Health at the School of Medicine, Yale University. He is the author and co-author of over 450 publications on the processes of recovery from and in serious mental illnesses and addictions and the development and evaluation of innovative policies and programs to promote the recovery and community inclusion of individuals with these conditions.

Part I.
Our Journey

1
Stigma, Meet Hope
Katherine Ponte

It can be a long, hard road to recovery. And recovery is not a cure. Recovery in mental illness is living a full and meaningful life.

The journey starts with hope. It can be very hard to find or regain it. Stigma often blocks the way.

But courage and strength can clear the way. With a whole lot of hope, love and support, recovery is possible, but only if you dare to dream it. The example of others can help show you the way.

This is where it started for me.

It started by suspecting, feeling that something was not right, but dismissing it, hoping it would pass. The stresses of social injustice, a sexual assault by a friend and classmate, academic stress, career issues, family illness, disappointments to myself and my family. Finally, a visit to university health services leads to a shocking diagnosis in just a few minutes. I didn't even know what bipolar was. Nobody took the time to explain it to me. Nobody cared about all of my triggers. They just gave me a label and some meds. Threats of forced medical leave. I was marginalized, isolated and withdrawn. I felt so alone, far from home on that big campus. All of that hard work to get here, all of my dreams, now I'm on the verge of losing it all. I felt so much blind angry denial.

Many years pass. Another crisis erupts – 911…the NYPD in my living room…treatment, more denial, refusal, medical non-compliance. My doctor tells me things will only get worse. She's unbelievably patronizing. Forget my prior goals and ambitions. I dreaded my appointments. She says to me, "you ARE bipolar roman numeral number 1". I've lost my identity, I'm a disorder, a statistical abnormality. My self-esteem is utterly crushed. But wasn't she supposed to help me get better? Confusion about who or what's to blame. Who can I trust? It brings a whole lot of heartache for me, for those that I love.

This disease is devasting and cruel; at its worst, it takes lives. It assaults my mind when I'm manic. I believe I'm a prophet, I make religious shrines, I trash my apartment, I run all over the streets of NYC recklessly, I break into a house of worship to pray, an arrest, a criminal record, my moral superiority wreaks havoc. I buy a house sight unseen. I brought a homeless man home for tea.

At my peak, I experience a massive manic episode in the heart of NYC, at one of the city's most popular tourist destinations—John Lennon's Imagine Mosaic in Central Park. I imagine a world without me or anyone else in it, the end. God made me the messenger. Why can't others see it too? I was trying to save the world, while others laughed and took pictures of me. Sirens sound. This is it. My husband explains that I'm sick. The ambulance picks me up just steps away. The EMS wraps me in a sheet from head to toe to contain me, to hide me. They say I'm a wild one.

My husband was shocked each and every time. How could I be so reckless, oblivious to the dangers, so completely and totally mad out of my mind? But, it all made sense to me at the time.

Delusional, psychotic, floridly manic is how they described it. Then came 1 Relapse, then 2, 3 and 4, many close calls. Locked up one, two, three times in the psych ward, it feels like a jail, you can't come and go, no sunlight, no fresh breezes, the guards, solitary confinement, you're comatose. The physical and chemical restraints make clear—you're locked up.

When will the relapses end? This is bipolar in all of its glory. How can I live with this? I was mortified by all that I had done. How could anyone possibly forgive me?

I withdraw further and further. Isolation deeply seeps in, takes hold, was my existence. Barely existing, hardly surviving, wishing I could just end it all like so many like me have done so before, but no I don't want that at all—I just want the pain and suffering to stop, I want to be me, the me before bipolar struck, I want my life back, a life. I just can't stop crying. Marital strain. Can I ever have kids? What kind of manic mother would I be? I threw it all away, it took away my dreams.

Unemployment. Dependency. People now expect far less of me and some nothing at all, now that I'm just mentally ill. I am a lawyer, I went to an Ivy league for this? I expected so much more. I never thought I would end up settling for so much less. What a big fall. Oh the burden, the guilt.

This treatment, that treatment. This med, that med. Zyprexa. Obesity. Seroquel. Sedation. Lithium diseased my parathyroids. The side effects make it hard to stay on the meds. Now everyone just thinks I'm lazy, see how fat I've become. They minimize my pain and suffering, dishearten, discourage me when they say, "can't you just get better, cheer up." Am I to blame? Am I trying hard enough? Do they really think I like being this way? - poked and prodded? Nothing seems to work. Will anything ever work? Why bother?

Maybe, I'm just unlucky in life. How could this happen to me, how did it get so bad? Why God? Why me? All hope is lost. All that remains is pain and suffering. I hate my life, I hate myself. Self-stigma—the most powerful, most dangerous stigma of all. You are your condition. Shame and embarrassment. This is the rest of your life. Nothing suggests otherwise. That's why I wanted to end it all.

And others. I can't let them see me this way. I'd rather not see them at all. My mother keeps insisting, persisting. She won't leave me alone. My spouse never lets up. They always fear the worst now, rarely the better. I've got everyone on high alert 24/7. I avoid and hide my symptoms as best as I can. If they really know how I'm feeling, that I'm struggling it will only mean more trouble for me, back to the psych ward. And why cause worry and all of that pity and sorrow? How can anyone possibly like me anyway. Maybe before, but not now, never again. I'm completely alone—alone even from myself.

It just keeps getting worse with no end in sight, but all of a sudden, out of the blue it starts to get just a little bit better. I see someone who's done it. Who's taken back their life, others fighting their way through it. I think maybe...maybe I can too. Stigma has kept me in exile for far too long. I've had enough. When hope finally returns, it takes stigma down.

I start to get back up on my feet. 1 step, 2 steps, 3 steps forward, 2 steps backwards, forward again. And so on. It's a slow journey. But it is doable. Despite what many may say, many may think, mental illness is not a terminal illness. I self-empower, l love myself, I take care of myself, most importantly I believe in myself, I believe I deserve so much more, I believe I can and I will get better. Others have done so and so can I.

Adding to that, more positive examples and a whole lot of love and support—a caring and loving family, great medical care all lifting my hope. I reach stability but that was not enough. I had to reach recovery to have a full and meaningful life. I reach it. I'm in recovery. I've arrived to where I hope will be the rest of my life.

It's a truly wonderful to be alive again - a family, a career, happiness. I am eager to show people the new me, to tell them, "I know what you thought about me, because I thought it too, but look at me now". I tell anyone and everyone who will listen to me that everything stigma said about me was just one big lie. I stand up to stigma by creating ForLikeMinds.com to help others like me overcome stigma to reach recovery. By allowing us to connect with each other, we can support and inform each other so we can pursue recovery together.

I return to the Imagine Mosaic nearly every day. Now, I imagine, I see a world with me in it, happiness.

That's what happened to me when stigma, met hope. Because hope can conquer stigma. Recovery is real.

Originally published in *Schizophrenia Bulletin*, Volume 45, Issue 6, Nov. 2019.

2
Me – and My Wife's Bipolar Diagnosis
Izzy Gonçalves

I came home to my world upside down. My apartment entrance had been blocked, and music was blaring deep within. I finally got inside and found my wife, Katherine, in a "possessed" state. It was surreal: there I was, calling 911 to get her help. Paramedics arrived with several police— standard procedure for a psych call - but I thought: "is this a medical emergency or an arrest?" Stigma already started to set in.

What started as a minimum 72-hour hold would end up being several weeks in the psych ward. My wife, still manic when I first saw her, hated me, blaming me for calling for help. Her bipolar I diagnosis was unacceptable to her, and when she couldn't deny her illness any longer, she said I contributed to it.

Besides the trauma of Katherine's manic episodes and the years of trying to figure out a new normal as a couple (thankfully a recovery we enjoy now), I was inadequately prepared for the ambush of my own reactions: the initial shock followed by deep feelings of resentment, guilt, and anger.

Some of these emotions were due to my own confusion and uncertainty in trying to find a way forward with my wife. There was also little support; I didn't know of any couples dealing with bipolar and thriving or living well.

Katherine blamed me for playing a part in her illness, and yet needed me to care for her. I couldn't get past my resentment for how she reacted toward me. I missed work to see clinicians and plan for her return, and while at work, I fought the distraction of wondering how she would be once home. I felt angry that I was making all these sacrifices that she didn't appreciate.

I also couldn't help feeling guilt. I didn't know what had caused her manic episode. Maybe it was something I did. But in fact, a lot had recently happened to explain the episode – a combination of family stress, work stress, and traumatic events. I hadn't known enough to make the connections.

Neither of us really thought very much about how the other was feeling, and it took us a long time to address and work through these issues after she left the hospital. We both felt loss, which we now know is "ambiguous loss." My wife was still "there," but she was not the same. We were still together, but this was not the family life we had envisioned.

I probably fixated more on my losses than hers. Truthfully, I felt like a bit of a victim and resented her even more.

I was always more focused on preventing another chaotic manic episode, but depression was the most pronounced part of her condition. She was inactive and no longer creative. She was no longer hopeful, and I was no longer hopeful for her. I, too, was depressed. Our communication suffered as we became hardened by the illness. We were without hope for years.

That was until Katherine took more control of her treatment. Up until then I had communicated directly with her then-doctor. But after she changed doctors and had her medications adjusted, she found strength and hope from peer support.

We slowly entered a recovery phase that I hadn't thought was possible. It wasn't the smoothest transition for us, but we are now partners in her treatment. I discovered that we can both live fuller lives and we can both have more control over bipolar disorder's uncertainties.

We reached a better place together, which reconciled our former hopes and dreams with the realities of her diagnosis. The ambiguous loss was not a real loss. We didn't lose our former life together; it is just a different life now, and potentially a more fulfilling one.

Originally published in *bpHope, bp Magazine*, Spring 2019.

Part II.
Self-recognition

3
Hope and Recovery
Professor Larry Davidson, Ph.D.,
School of Medicine, Yale University

What is hope?

Hope is a complex concept that has been defined in many different ways, especially within the context of mental health. Mental illnesses have been thought of as disorders of time in which a person's past, present, and future become disconnected from each other (Schrank, Hayward, Stanghellini, & Davidson, 2011). In this view, hope is conceived of as a thread that reconnects and reunifies past, present, and future, enabling people to find new meanings in their past and to imagine a better future for themselves. Hope is thus considered necessary for recovery from mental illness (Schrank et al., 2011). For example, remembering how one overcame difficulties in the past can ignite hope for the present and future (Darlington & Bland, 1999).

In the health research literature, hope has been variously defined as an emotion (i.e., the desire for something positive to happen and the feeling that this is possible); as a cognition or thought (i.e., thinking that reaching a desired goal or outcome is possible or likely), or as a combination of both (i.e., thinking that a desired outcome is possible and subsequently feeling positive emotions). Recently, a more multidimensional definition of hope has been proposed that also includes the notions of time (past experience and future desires), goals, control (through personal activity and/or environmental or contextual factors), relations, personal characteristics (inner strength, motivation, etc.), reality reference (the perception that desired outcomes are possible), and the notion that hope can spring from both satisfactory and unsatisfactory circumstances (Schrank et al., 2011).

Hope is pivotal to recovery

Research suggests that hope is crucial to recovery for persons with mental illness. A scoping review of research on the experience of hope among people with co-occurring mental health and substance use problems (Tore Saelor, Ness, Holgersen, & Davidson, 2014) found that hope was perceived as a facilitator of change and recovery, making change and getting better seem possible. Mental health professionals were seen to play a role in strengthening hope among service users by giving positive feedback and by simply being present. Importantly, *lack of hope* and unrealized expectations were cited as reasons for using substances, while *having hope* was cited as a reason for abstinence (Tore Saelor et al., 2014).

In another study, eight sessions of "hope therapy" offered to individuals with and without mental health conditions in which they were taught skills in goal-setting, planning to meet goals, finding sources of motivation, and monitoring progress resulted in increased feelings of agency, suggesting that teaching individuals how to have hope can be a step towards recovery (Schrank et al., 2011).

The hope that is sparked by peer support services and the experience of meeting peers recovering from mental illness has also been described as playing "an early, and often crucial, role in promoting recovery" (Schrank et al., 2011, p. 15).

Sources of hope and how it can be fostered

When a person with a mental illness is feeling hopeless and discouraged, simply having someone else believe in them and have hope *for* them can be a powerful source of hope. Patricia Deegan, one of the early leaders of the mental health consumer/survivor movement, termed this "surrogate hope" (Schrank et al., 2011) because this hope is held *for you* by another person. Persons holding this surrogate hope can in turn be thought of as "hope carriers" (Darlington & Bland, 1999). For instance, clinicians having genuine confidence in a person's ability to recover and explicitly conveying this hope to them by communicating the possibility, and indeed, the probability, of recovery, can instill hope or at least sustain a person until they are able to develop hope for themselves.

To do this, however, clinicians must move beyond the traditional focus on deficits and disorder to embrace the whole person: that is, as someone having strengths, interests, resilience, and aspirations that can be actively fostered and supported (Schrank et al., 2011; Tore Sælør et al., 2014; Darlington & Bland, 1999). By asking about a person's aspirations and life dreams, recognizing and helping develop their strengths, and connecting them to opportunities to realize these, clinicians, family members, and others supporting persons with mental illnesses can help cultivate hope. It is also important that supporters work within a person's frame of reference (Darlington & Bland, 1999), not imposing hope on them and being realistic by grounding hope in the person's own experiences and abilities. For example, when supporters acknowledge individuals' small gains and improvements, and remind them of their past gains and successful strategies for overcoming difficulty, they can promote hope (Darlington & Bland, 1999).

Users of mental health services have expressed that being helped to understand their condition can impart hope, as this knowledge empowers them (e.g., to seek help when symptoms worsen) and helps them reclaim control. More fundamentally, both service users and clinicians feel that clinicians being genuine and human, treating service users as regular people, and truly believing in their capacity to get better are essential qualities that promote hope (Darlington & Bland, 1999).

When one is resigned to a lackluster life, the unexpected experience of simple pleasures can also spark hope, reminding individuals with mental illness of the possibilities for a rewarding and meaningful life. This hope is required for individuals to take the risks necessary for recovery and growth (Schrank et al., 2011).

Finally, peer support services are uniquely placed to inspire hope by providing living models of recovery, as peer support workers literally embody the hope of recovery. Seeing someone who has had similar experiences and made it through can be an incredibly strong source of hope for individuals with mental illnesses who are in despair and feeling alone in their experience (Schrank et al., 2011).

Conclusions

Hope is critically important, particularly for persons with mental illnesses, but also for their clinicians, families, and others who offer them support. Despite evidence for the importance of hope in recovery, the concept of hope remains difficult to define and research on the topic is scarce (Tore Sælør et al., 2014). There is a need for more research exploring firsthand experiences of hope among persons with mental illnesses so that we can better understand how it is subjectively defined and experienced and what inspires it (Tore Saelor et al., 2014). That being said, the evidence to date suggests that peer support and strengths-based clinical practices are promising ways to instill hope and promote recovery.

Larry Davidson, Ph.D. is a Professor of Psychiatry and Director of the Program for Recovery and Community Health at the School of Medicine, Yale University. He is the author and co-author of over 450 publications on the processes of recovery from and in serious mental illnesses and addictions and the development and evaluation of innovative policies and programs to promote the recovery and community inclusion of individuals with these conditions.

References

Darlington, Y., & Bland, R. (1999). Strategies for encouraging and maintaining hope among people living with serious mental illness. *Australian Social Work, 52*(3), 17-23.

Schrank, B., Hayward, M., Stanghellini, G., & Davidson, L. (2011). Hope in psychiatry. *Advances in Psychiatric Treatment, 17*(3), 227-235.

Tore Saelor, K., Ness, O., Holgersen, H., & Davidson, L. (2014). Hope and recovery: a scoping review. *Advances in Dual Diagnosis, 7*(2), 63-72.

Originally published in *ForLikeMinds Evidence*, 2019.

4
Power to Create Change
Comes from Within
Katherine Ponte

Stigma is a shield created by society, made up of misunderstanding and fear of mental illness. When we look away from someone behaving erratically or "strangely" on the street, that's the fear society ingrains in us. Perhaps we're scared to consider the possibility that the same could happen to us, that we might be shunned by society too.

The shield of stigma also stops us from seeking help for our own mental health. When faced with a stressful life event or emotional challenges, we might carry the hurt or confusion inside. Perhaps we avoid facing a potential diagnosis, so our illness only grows worse. Stigma facilitates mental illness turning into the "monster" it doesn't have to be.

Social perceptions need to change. However, stigma is so deeply rooted in societal norms that it can take a long time to eradicate. And people like me, people living with mental illness, can't wait on society to change. We need to live now. In fact, we need to be pioneers.

Our Experience Combats Stigma

First, we need to overcome our own belief in society's fears. This requires finding hope, and specifically recognizing the possibility of recovery. Recovery from mental illness is living a full and productive life with mental illness. With this mindset, we can take ownership of our condition and live a fulfilling life. This can be one of the most powerful forces for change.

Stories of living fully with mental illness can help reshape society's bias. They also provide inspiration and guidance for other people living with mental illness. This is the power of peer support and sharing lived experience. It creates a cycle of more people finding recovery, and then in turn, society seeing more positive examples of people living well with mental illness. Society needs to see what life with mental illness can and should be - a life of possibility, not a life sentence.

Our Experience Inspires Others

When people share their mental health journeys, it also helps set our own expectations. Recovery is hard, and there is no smooth path to get there. It's also not a cure, it requires continuous patience, discipline and determination. There will be stumbles and uncertainties along the way. This is the reality of mental illness. That's why relatable, real-life examples are so valuable.

Knowing that others are going through similar challenges can help us build resilience. The result is self-empowerment by the example of others. We, the mental health community, rely less on the image society projects upon us, and instead focus on the image reflected to us by our peers. This is the power from within ourselves and our community.

I believe that this type of person-driven recovery has been overlooked as a way to combat social stigma. It's become so ingrained that not even people with mental illness think recovery is possible. Too many of us allow society's fears to become our own. Together, we can reverse the vicious cycle of stigma and instead, power the virtuous cycle of hope and recovery.

Originally published in *National Alliance on Mental Illness National Blog*, Oct. 24, 2018.

5
Two Antidotes to Stigma
Katherine Ponte

Stigma had a lot to say about me. "She's bipolar. She'll always be sick. She can't function normally, work, make decisions or take risks." It reduced me to a child. It destroyed my self-esteem and self-worth. It made me feel hopeless and helpless. Because of this, I refused my diagnosis, help and treatment. I lost a lot of years to it – not to the illness itself, but to the struggle with stigma.

Stigma can be harshest for those of us who experience psychosis. Society often views us and portrays us to be the most dangerous, unpredictable and least likely to recover. We are often the scapegoat for social ills like gun violence. We are sensationalized and generalized in the media. It makes us feel alienated and misunderstood.

Even some doctors hold stigmatizing views against those of us with severe mental illness. The most damaging stigma I ever encountered was when my past doctor told me, "your bipolar will only get worse." I was left without hope. I had no say in my care. She gave me no respect. I was treated like a disease, not a person. She said to me "you are bipolar roman numeral one." It is devastating to feel stigma from the person who is supposed to help you get better.

Thankfully I'm in recovery now. My current psychiatrist does not make me feel stigmatized. He respects me and lets me have a say in my care. Stigma harms me less, but I still must remain vigilant. My experience has shown me many forms of stigma and how to fight against it. Here are the two ways I believe are the most effective.

Coming Out with Our Diagnosis

I'm in recovery now thanks to someone's brave act of coming out. While in the hospital, I learned of a woman living with schizophrenia who shared her own message of recovery with the public. I was shocked. I never knew recovery was possible until I saw her. All along stigma told me this could never happen to me. In an instant, her message inspired me, it sparked my hope that had long been dormant. It motivated me to work as hard as I could to reach recovery.

Our self-esteem and self-efficacy have been battered by stigma, but it can be restored by coming out. We should not be ashamed nor afraid. By coming out, we can connect with each other and people who don't understand mental illness. We can show them that we are wonderful people, not much different from them. We can replace their discomfort, distrust and fear with empathy and compassion. We can replace myths and stereotypes with facts, let others know that mental illness can be treated and managed. It is the most effective anti-stigma approach.

We need campaigns that spread these peer examples. We can't wait for recovery to come to us. Countless people living with mental illness can benefit from the relatable examples of others living with mental illness whether those peers are struggling or well.

Sadly, coming out is not an option for many, due to personal circumstances and stigma's many potential adverse consequences for basic human needs like well-paying jobs, safe housing and quality health care. Some may benefit greatly as I did, some may not. It's a deeply personal and private matter. And once you're out, you're out. We must all think carefully about disclosing our diagnoses, and online resources can even help with the process. However, part of this decision is understanding the potential positive impact we can have.

The impact of peer examples on me was so profound that it inspired me to come out, even with one of the most stigmatized conditions – severe bipolar I disorder with psychosis. Sharing my experience furthered my recovery by increasing my sense of self-empowerment, self-esteem, self-worth and support from others. By inspiring and supporting others, coming out will also contribute to combating stigma in our society. My impact compounds as it influences others to share their stories, who then influence others, and so on.

Leading Our Community

The mental health community is large. However, very few of our leaders have a condition themselves. Many leaders of organizations representing people with mental illness have seen it firsthand through a friend or a relative who has mental illness. But knowing someone who has mental illness and having mental illness are not the same.

Only we know what it's like to live with mental illness. We know our wants and needs best. Our mental health system would be much better if we were more involved. But again, stigma has prevented us from coming forward and representing ourselves. And staying out of the important conversations only perpetuates and intensifies certain stigmas about people with mental illness.

We need to speak more for ourselves. We need to assume our power and pursue our goals. We welcome and value the respectful guidance and counsel of our allies, but we need to increasingly lead the way in advocating for and supporting our community. We are at our most powerful when we're standing together.

I wish many things for my community that I love very dearly. Sadly, our history is filled with cruel and dehumanizing treatment. Once we were cast off by society – discarded in asylums, locked up, isolated, immobilized, even lobotomized and sterilized. Now, many of our peers are in jails and prisons or living in extreme poverty on the streets. We must not let stigma silence the cries of our community to allow these wrongs to continue. We must advocate for each other.

I wish all people with mental illness, whether we're struggling or well, will be accepted, respected and fairly treated. It's time for individual and social change that recognizes our humanity. We are capable of recovery. We can and should have full and meaningful lives.

Originally published in *National Alliance on Mental Illness National Blog*, Feb. 3, 2020.

6
Embracing the Diversity within Us
Katherine Ponte

Everybody has multiple identities whether or not they're living with mental illness. Among those most important to me: I am a kind-hearted person, a wife, a daughter, a friend, a volunteer, an entrepreneur, a Portuguese-Canadian-American, a Catholic, an Ivy League graduate, and I happen to be a person living with mental illness.

All of this and much more is me. I am proud of all of me. The many aspects of my identity greatly enhance who I am. They give me multiple sources of strength to draw on which help me cope with the challenges of mental illness.

In order for our identities to promote mental health, we have to let ourselves be empowered by them. In particular, a person's identities can enhance their sense of belonging because they can allow membership and connection with multiple communities. This can be particularly helpful to mental health.

Our Identity Can Enhance Our Mental Health

I live my life, day-by-day, with the goal of spreading kindness and see this as a large part of my identity. Performing acts of kindness makes me extremely happy. It's sometimes known as the helper's high and shows the positive impact of helping others. I am very fortunate that I am able to intertwine my volunteer and work activities, which brings me immense pleasure that also triggers a helper's high. The "community service" nature of much of my work compensates me in ways far beyond economic gain.

I was born and raised Catholic. My religious beliefs and practices have provided very effective coping strategies for me, such as meditation in the form of prayer. There are many potential mental health benefits of religion and spirituality. These include gaining a framework for understanding the meaning of life and inclusion in a faith community.

I am Portuguese-Canadian-American. I love the "small village life" in Portugal's rural communities. I love that in Canada medical care is accessible to all. I love America's dogged determination to overcome any challenge. This "ethnic pride" protects my mental health. I celebrate all of my ethnicities, cultures and traditions. They are a source of both emotional strength and protection.

I proudly consider having a mental illness as one of my identities. There is no community that I could possibly be prouder of. My recovery journey is the greatest challenge of my life. It tested me, it brought out my courage and strength, my resilience. It made me more empathetic and compassionate.

Our Identity is Multi-dimensional

"We cannot separate the importance of a sense of belonging from our physical and mental health." Lacking a sense of belonging can lead to depression, anxiety and suicide. One study of people living with schizophrenia found that they considered a sense of belonging vital, yet they more frequently felt isolated and/or like they didn't belong. Even the smallest social belonging interventions can yield lasting positive effects.

Unfortunately, stigma prevents many people from viewing themselves fully enough to recognize their belonging and sources of strength from multiple identities. In many cases, when a person develops a mental illness, their diminished self-worth and self-stigma leads them to *only* identify as a person living with mental illness.

Families often reinforce this belief by focusing on a person's mental illness as their primary reason for engagement. Society reinforces the concept as well with damaging stereotypes. Stigma can also make it impossible to realize the basic, most important identities we develop through our interactions with others — to be accepted, to belong and to contribute. Therefore, due to stigma, a person living with mental illness may be regarded to hold a "socially devalued role," which can make it extremely difficult to reach recovery.

By ignoring a person's multiple identities, this narrow-minded view ignores a person's many sources of strength and value. It ignores the social roles that give a person meaning and purpose.

The social role valorization (SRV) model seeks to make it easier for socially devalued people to obtain the "good things in life," such as family and friends, community and work, among many others. The SRV model helps place socially devalued people into a role of social value by using "culturally valued means to enable, establish, enhance, maintain, and/or defend valued social roles for people at value risk." *The Keys to a Good Life Handbook* provides a good overview.

Our Identity is Our Strength

I will not let people define me by my mental illness *alone*. I'll proudly and adamantly assert that my mental illness is a part of who I am, an important part. Our mental illness community needs a whole lot more pride, self-esteem and self-worth. We need to love ourselves and accept the love of others, because we deserve it.

In the end, it is of course up to each person to decide how to identify themselves. But many parts of our identities can be sources of untapped strength that can help us cope with the challenges of living with mental illness.

References

The Keys to a Good Life Handbook provides a good overview.
https://adobe.ly/3dsN7rR

Originally published in *National Alliance on Mental Illness Blog*, Jul. 8, 2020.

7
The Stages of My Mental Illness
Katherine Ponte

I was conditioned to view my illness on a scale of "severe" to "less severe." I was accustomed to doctors describing my condition based on how I was doing *at that moment* rather than where I was on my mental health journey. This approach echoes exactly what's wrong with the way we approach mental illness - as a permanent state rather than a path towards living well. In fact, for too many years, doctors didn't even tell me about the prospect of recovery.

When I started feeling better, I realized that mental illness is a process. And I believe that approaching mental illness as a process and a journey to recovery can foster hope and improve treatment outcomes. It can also help loved ones understand and participate in the recovery experience.

The following are the steps I took on my mental illness journey, along with what helped me or what would have helped me. I hope they help others chart their own path to recovery.

Symptom Onset and Diagnosis

At the time of my symptom onset and diagnosis, I was experiencing intense academic pressure, career uncertainties, family illness and trauma from a sexual assault. I was convinced that these experiences were the cause of my distress and I wish someone had validated these emotions. I managed to see a psychiatrist, but they seemed more interested in putting a label on me than seeing me as a whole person.

A more empathetic, compassionate and informative initial doctor visit would have definitely helped. The first visit is critical—it strongly influences diagnosis acceptance and follow-up care. I also wish I had brought friends or family to support me. Without these things, I dismissed my diagnosis and it went untreated for many years.

Crisis

Ultimately, I had a crisis—a full manic episode. I was forcibly taken from my home under police escort and was hospitalized. I was angry at my spouse for making that 911-call. But afterwards, we were both relieved it was seemingly over. No one discussed the likelihood of a relapse. So we were both unprepared when my spouse had to call 911 again in the coming years.

I wish my psychiatrist had carefully and realistically discussed the possibility of relapse and what we should do in a crisis situation. Only after my third hospitalization did my spouse and I talk about the potential for future episodes. Discussing it at a time of calm and stability allowed us to develop a crisis plan without pressure and with clarity of mind. Having a plan has provided both of us with some sense of ownership in the treatment process.

Withdrawal and Isolation

I withdrew and isolated after my diagnosis and hospitalizations. I didn't want to talk about them, didn't know how to talk about them, and I didn't want to be a burden on my loved ones. This was very difficult for my mom. She would call me, but I refused to speak or said very little.

My mom learned how to communicate with me when I was isolating. She stopped asking me how I was doing; instead she would text me, "I hope you're okay," which was better. She also started sending me small, loving gifts. The gifts really meant a lot to me when I was very ill. In fact, they were the inspiration for RecoveryBoosters, my gift shop for people with depression. Eventually, my mom expressed that the single most important thing to her was to receive a nightly text telling her I had taken my medications—so I still do that to this day.

Treatment

My spouse did everything he could to get me the right treatment. When I was unhappy with my first psychiatrist, he found me another one. Initially, I was hopeful and optimistic with the change, but my spouse and doctor started communicating directly and making treatment decisions for me. I felt completely disempowered and excluded from my own care.

When I moved on to my third psychiatrist, I took full ownership and control of my treatment, and the outcomes were far better. My spouse saw me improve and learned to respect my need to control my own care. I didn't want to exclude him; I just wanted to be directly involved too. We reached an agreement on when and how he can contact my doctor. We even developed a Collaborative Care Plan (see Appendix I. Additional Resources) as a tool for improving interactions among families and with clinicians.

Stability and Recovery

For many years, I struggled to reach and stay in stability. I think I struggled as much as I did because I wasn't satisfied with stability being my end-goal. My treatment seemed solely focused on not being combative, in a crisis, hypomanic or manic. The cost of this was not living fully. Stability meant surviving, but not thriving. This was not the life I wanted to live. I needed so much more.

Recovery is about experiencing. It's about pursuing. It's about thriving. It's about living fully. Recovery is about managing risks, the risks we all need to take to achieve our best selves. After I learned of recovery, I was filled with uncontrollable anticipation, but I realized that I needed stability to pursue it. I needed stability as a transition not an end-goal. Recovery could be on the other side.

Stability and recovery would not have been possible without the love and support of my spouse. He enabled the most important part of my recovery—the ability to dream and pursue my dreams.

I knew I had reached recovery when I felt ready to fulfill my dream of helping others by creating ForLikeMinds. For over 15 years, I was afraid to dream because I was convinced that I would be disappointed. But my doctors, spouse and I are working together to maintain my health.

My journey from that first diagnosis to recovery has been long and hard, full of pain and suffering for me and my loved ones. That journey is never-ending—there is no cure for bipolar. But now, my family's support helps guide the way along familiar roads I've traveled before. They make the journey less uncertain, more manageable, more endurable because I know this is the way to continued recovery.

Originally published in *National Alliance on Mental Illness Blog*, Nov. 7, 2018.

8
Addressing Emotions with Mental Illness
Katherine Ponte

People with mental illness experience a wide range of emotions. My caregiver and I were not prepared for the emotional onslaught my bipolar triggered. For me, the three most prominent emotions were anger, lack of self-worth and, eventually, hope. They reflect my evolution from mental illness diagnosis towards recovery.

Stigma leads may people to think those of us with mental illness cannot control our emotions, that we are "overly emotional" or "moody." This created a significant obstacle for me to accept and discuss my mental illness. Peer support allowed me to take that first step.

We all experience emotions differently for many reasons, but I hope this piece can help others living with mental illness and their loved ones better understand and address their emotions.

My Experience with Anger

The most difficult emotion to manage can be resentment, anger or rage according to the many people I've consulted through my recovery coaching service. This was also true for my spouse and me. My anger, as often is the case, was based in fear. I feared that I would lose the life I had. I felt a fear of abandonment by friends and family for many years.

I sometimes unreasonably took out my anger on my spouse. I blamed him for my illness. He thought I hated and resented him. At times, he seemed more focused on what he was experiencing than what I was experiencing. He said hurtful things. I said hurtful things. I now know that I wasn't angry at him. I was angry at the illness, at my situation. We were hurting, and we hurt each other more. It was a vicious cycle.

What I Learned

Because my illness monopolized our conversations, I felt like I had ceased to be a person. I was merely a disease. Our relationship felt like a side note or a circumstance in which the disease existed. It's important to realize that a relationship may need treatment too. Actively managing and nurturing the relationship, sometimes through formal counseling during times of struggle, can positively influence treatment outcomes.

Focusing on recovery as a common goal can bring a family dealing with mental illness closer together. As we focused on treating our relationship, my spouse recognized the underlying roots of my anger and adjusted his approach. He insisted that I play a greater role in my care instead of letting me depend on him. He grew to respect and trust my concerns. His role changed from that of guardian to protect me from myself to a partner in a Collaborative Care Plan (see Appendix I. Additional Resources). It made all the difference.

I had imagined my spouse much better off in a "normal" relationship. Deep down, I knew that he was deeply committed to me, but I needed to hear it repeatedly. That affirmation can be very valuable. A sense of stability and belonging can be critical to good mental health.

My Experience with Lack of Self-Worth

Not too far along into my illness, I lost all self-worth. I felt like a loser and a failure. I was hypersensitive. I felt mental illness had taken away my intelligence, even neutralized my degrees. I grieved my former self, which I believed I could never return to. I felt like a disappointment to my friends and family. I felt unloved, and worse, unlovable.

I suffered from extreme self-stigma, which led to suicidal ideation and an extended period of deep depression. I would isolate and withdraw completely. I was at times unable to get out of bed. I cancelled appointments. I missed exams. I refused all attempts by others to connect with me. Sleeping was my only escape.

What I Learned

Mental illness can make a person feel profoundly changed, and it's important for caregivers to be aware of that. The shame we feel is often related to how we think we make our loved ones feel. I was deeply saddened when people in my life would say things like "you used to be so…" as it only reinforced my own insecurities and grief.

Loved ones should avoid these types of statements. For many with mental illness, we desperately want our families to view us in the same way they did before we got sick. Caregivers should reject when we say we're failures. They can also remind us of challenges we've overcome. Caregivers should validate our grief by giving hope, saying things like "I know that it's a difficult time right now, but things will get better. These are only temporary setbacks."

At my lows, I did not feel worthy of friendships. I had a wonderful friend, Nuno, at the time. Nuno refused to let me isolate and withdraw. Every few days, he'd appear at my doorstep and knock until I responded. After exhausting all my excuses, we'd go out to lunch or dinner. I'd want to talk about how I was feeling. He'd listen attentively and then change the topic. All of this helped. He never stopped coming.

Nuno is the sort of friend every person with mental illness needs. Sometimes we do not want to go out with others because we don't believe they really want to be with us. And some of our friends may not connect with us simply because they don't know what to say. But you don't even have to talk about the illness. Just be there.

My Experience with Hope

For nearly 15 years living with mental illness, my hope was fleeting. A new medication would spark hope, but a failed attempt would take it all away. I sunk deeper and deeper into depression with every failed attempt. Hope can be complicated. You yearn for it, but you fear the anguish of disappointment.

Suddenly, unexpectedly, my hope was rekindled during a low point, my last hospitalization. A 10-minute video of a woman living with serious mental illness sparked it. Hope came rushing back and filled my heart with enough courage and determination to commit to recovery. The difference this time was that I saw that recovery was possible, and that it required my active involvement in treatment. It was the tiniest spark of hope that led me to recovery.

What I Learned

An enduring sense of hope is the most powerful emotion of all. It can be the key to recovery. How we experience hope will vary. It can come in many forms: rebirth, confidence, ownership, responsibility, commitment, trust, discipline, self-worth, excitement, optimism, self-determination, aspiration, energy or pride. Any of these emotions can lead to recovery.

The greatest challenge is finding the spark, which may require repeated and creative attempts.

It can be overwhelming to manage hope once you've rediscovered it. Many people living with mental illness who experience a "rebirth" want to make up for lost time. Careful goal-setting and execution is important to build on progress and minimize setbacks.

A SMART Goals (see resources) approach can be extremely helpful in managing goals and expectations. For example, experiencing hope of recovery may not quickly lead to starting a new job or career. Hope grows with the accomplishment of each goal. Caregivers should acknowledge and praise new efforts. Good medical treatment and supportive relationships can sustain and support hope towards recovery.

As a recovery coach, the key piece of advice I offer my clients is that they should address the emotions their mental illness triggers first. Otherwise, negative emotions will get in the way of treatment. If you embrace your emotions, and seek to understand them, it can improve both your relationships with others and your relationship with yourself.

Originally published in *National Alliance on Mental Illness Blog*, May 15, 2020.

9
Talking about Mental Illness: Reaching In
Katherine Ponte

Social support plays a key role in mental health and mental illness recovery. Tapping this support sooner would have accelerated my own recovery. Getting support starts with talking about our mental health. But friends and family shouldn't just wait for their loved one struggling with mental health to reach out.

When you "reach in" to your loved one, it not only helps them, it also breaks through the communication barriers often created by stigma. Talking about mental illness requires thoughtfulness, but it's not as hard as people may think. There is no universal way to talk about mental illness, but there are best practices that can help supporters start the conversation.

A Few General Best Practices

The following strategies might help set the right tone for communicating with your loved one.

Learn more first

Supporters often don't know what to say in the first talk. Knowing a little about mental health can help. This may include learning basics like emotions, symptoms and treatment modalities from reliable sources, such as NAMI.

Watch out for stigma

Always be aware of stigma, which includes self-stigma and perceived stigma. Remember and emphasize that mental illness is a lot like physical illness and is not their fault. Also, try not to talk to your loved one any differently than before they got sick.

Encourage

The key is to listen more and talk less. Ask open-ended questions to encourage them to share more. Emphasize their strengths and validate their emotions, which will make them feel more comfortable talking to you and opening up.

Offer support and empathy

Provide support and informed guidance, not advice. When it comes to mental illness, advice should come from mental health professionals. It may be counter-productive coming from a supporter. Additionally, offer empathy and compassion, not sympathy. To understand the difference, see a great YouTube video called Brené Brown on Empathy.

Meet us "where we're at"

When addressing mental illness, ask your loved one if they're comfortable discussing it and respect their wishes. Some of us just need more time to process our illness. Let us know that you're there whenever we want to talk and gently check in from time to time.

The First Talk

An initial discussion may be the most important so plan and prepare accordingly. These suggestions may help.

- If possible, talk to your loved one while they are well. It can help minimize adverse reactions and they will be able to give guidance on how to be supportive when they are not well.

- Normalize the conversation. Personally, I feel a casual talk can relieve pressure and make it easier on both sides.

- Prepare for varied and sometimes unpredictable reactions. Many people are ashamed and embarrassed about their illness. They may be angry or hopeless.

- If they refuse to talk, gently nudge them. It they continue to resist, stop and respect their privacy. A loved one may respond very angrily if they feel pressured.

- If the first conversation goes poorly, which is common, don't be afraid to try again at a later time.

What to Say and What Not to Say

While supporters act out of love and care, how they communicate affects how their loved one perceives their true intentions and feelings. The following dos and don'ts may help strike the right tone.

Be sensitive

Don't say: I have to talk to you.

Say: I noticed that you have not been sleeping or eating as much lately, would you like to talk about it?

Don't say: This has to stop.

Say: How can I help you feel better?

Don't say: It's your fault.

Say: Mental illness can happen to anyone.

Don't say: It's all in your head. It's not really that bad.

Say: I noticed that you haven't been yourself lately, would you like to talk about it?

Don't say: You need to [...].

Say: Can you tell me how you're feeling and how I can help?

Avoid stigma

Don't say: You are bipolar.

Say: You are a person with bipolar (always use person-first language).

Don't say: Stop acting crazy.

Say: You don't seem like yourself lately. Would you like to talk about it?

Don't say: You're just lazy.

Say: I know that you're not feeling well and that must make it hard for you to do things.

Cooperate

Don't say: You have to see a doctor

Say: I can't say for certain, but a doctor might be able to help you. Would you like to look for one together? I can go to an appointment with you.

Don't say: You need to focus on getting better.

Say: We can get through this together.

Encourage

Don't say: This is your life now, and you have to accept it.

Say: I have seen examples of people with mental illness living full lives. Things can get better. I will help any way I can.

Don't say: You're not getting better. Why doesn't therapy work?

Say: Mental illness can be managed and treated, sometimes it just takes finding the right treatment team and plan. I'll help you as much as I can.

Special Cases to Consider

With mental illness, there are certain situations that may need to be addressed in a more specific way.

Refusal / Resistance

Some of the most difficult conversations involve accepting diagnosis and treatment. In these cases, applying a strategy called LEAP by Dr. Xavier Amador can be very effective. LEAP is an acronym for:

- Listen. Use reflective listening to understand what your loved one feels, wants and believes without commenting, disagreeing or arguing.

- Empathize with your loved one's reasons to resist talking taking action, even those you disagree with.

- Agree. Look for common ground and acknowledge that your loved one has personal choice and responsibility.

- Partner to accomplish common goals.

Suicidal Behavior

It is important to talk openly about suicidal behavior, including suicidal ideation. Studies have found that "acknowledging and talking about suicide may in fact reduce, rather than increase suicidal ideation, and may lead to improvements in mental health in treatment-seeking populations," contrary to popular belief.

All conversations about suicide must be taken seriously. Never promise to keep the conversation confidential. The website Speaking of Suicide is a great resource and Living Works also offers a two-day Suicide Intervention Skills Trainings (ASIST) across the country.

After the First Talk

It is important to continue to engage your loved one after raising the topic as mental illness is an ongoing experience. "Talking" can happen through many modes. Initially, I preferred to talk by text. It was easier for my mom to share a sentiment without me getting defensive or risking an argument.

When I was saddest, I'd love "emoji text" exchanges without words — they showed me that my mom was thinking of me and showed my mom that I was well enough to text her back. She would also send me cards and flowers, which I always loved. All this made it easier for me to open up to my mom when I started to feel better. Sometimes not talking, just listening, just being there, can be really helpful.

Talking about mental illness can be difficult. Sometimes it requires repeated or creative attempts. These attempts may result in disappointments and feelings of frustration, helplessness or worry, but supporters should keep trying.

The more a supporter tries, the more likely it is for their loved one to truly understand how much they are loved, which is a powerful force. It can be the single most important factor in getting a person with mental illness to open up. Your patience and endurance will show them the truth and allow them to get the care that they need.

Originally published in *National Alliance on Mental Illness Blog*, May 20, 2020.

10
Coming Out about Your Bipolar Disorder
Katherine Ponte

The decision to disclose your diagnosis of bipolar disorder is very difficult. Here is everything you need to know before you go public.

When it comes to sharing your diagnosis of bipolar disorder, coming out is hard to do, but it may be the best thing for you. I stayed "closeted" about my mental health condition for over ten years, but my bipolar and the inexplicable unusual behavior that came with it outed me many times. I hoped and prayed that people might think I was having a bad day when I behaved erratically, but that was likely wishful thinking. I started to wonder if disclosing my diagnosis might actually benefit me. I weighed the pros and cons. The pros won.

Here are some of the pros for me:

- Reconnecting – Staying in the closet made me lonely. Coming out and no longer being ashamed and embarrassed allowed me to once again reconnect with people. I could engage with people I knew and also develop new relationships, especially with those who are also living with mental health conditions. I was able to volunteer to help this community. I surrounded myself with a "safe community" that I knew wouldn't stigmatize me.

- Feeling proud of who I am – I wanted to show people that I was proud of who I was. Even if bipolar was part of me, it was not all of me. I refused to let my mental health condition define me as I had for so many years. Coming out actually made me stronger. It was empowering to take control of my health and life. I also grew to appreciate how empathetic and compassionate our community is.

- Not living a lie – I was tired of pretending that I was well when I wasn't. I wanted my friends and family to better understand mental health conditions like mine. By being honest I could promote greater understanding.

- Being able to apologize – I wanted to apologize to the people I had hurt while ill. My bipolar caused me to hurt people unintentionally, by my words and my actions. I wanted to apologize; I wanted to relieve myself of the burden of guilt I carried for so long. I wanted people to understand that my actions were not intentional. Most were compassionate, and our friendships grew stronger.

- Growing my support network – Staying in the closet cut me off from a lot of my friends. I wanted to reconnect with them honestly and genuinely. I wanted them to know all of me, the real me. Disclosing my diagnosis also allowed me to include people with mental health conditions in my support network. That was very helpful because we could relate to each other's experiences. Also, some of the friends I came out to shared that they lived with mental health conditions, too. It made me feel less alone.

- Support network for my supporters – I wanted my supporters to also grow their own support network. For a long time, I forbid my mother and father from ever telling anyone I had bipolar. That cut my mom off from sharing those caregiver experiences with others. In doing so, she could not get the support she also needed. I gave my mom permission to disclose my mental health condition to her close friends; as a result, she was able to receive more support. Supporters need support, too.

- Rejoining the family – I missed too many family get-togethers because of my bipolar. I was afraid that people could tell just by looking at me that something was wrong with me. I was afraid I might ruin the festive event we had gathered for. I was afraid that I might embarrass my mom and dad. I wanted my family dinners, holidays, and reunions back, and I was tired of "fake smiling" when I attended or being "sick with a cold" at home when I wasn't up to attending.

- Setting an example for others – And perhaps most importantly, I wanted to set an example for other people living with mental health conditions. I hoped to encourage them not to be embarrassed and ashamed as I had been for so long. I wanted to show them that stability is possible, and I hoped that my story would inspire hope. Over time, as I developed ForLikeMinds, I recognized increasingly the opportunity to educate people about mental health.

Inspirational examples helped motivate me to come out

I was really inspired by LGBTQ+ coming out stories. Their courage and bravery in both coming out and facing the risks to their mental health were motivating. I have heard of many people who identify as part of the LGBTQ+ community experiencing depression and anxiety over the coming out process. I love that there is a National Coming Out Day for the LGBTQ+ community. It's a day when they harness their collective courage to provide the support of the community to members who are coming out. This act of unification really inspired me. I wish the mental health community had its own coming out day.

I was also of course inspired by the examples of other people living with mental illness who also decided to come out. It is invaluable to know that others have done so successfully and were so much better off for it. Their example made me feel that my own coming out would work out.

Whom to come out to first:

- Close friends – they can support you when you come out to others. If your close friends are truly close friends, you shouldn't lose them. I didn't lose mine.

- Other friends – expect to lose some. And if you do, they're not worth keeping. I love that quote attributed to Dr. Seuss: "Those who matter don't mind, and those who mind don't matter."

- Relatives – you may want your parents or other close family to share the news with your other relatives. We may actually care about what these relatives think. If they react with insensitivity, or, worse, with negativity, we may actually be hurt by their reaction, so your parents or close family can serve as a buffer.

- Social colleagues, casual acquaintances – I didn't come out to them at first. I assess if they may be a good source of support as I learn more about them and our relationship develops.

- Work colleagues – This is possibly the riskiest group to come out to. Employers may ignorantly fear that people with mental health conditions are less productive, have diminished mental capacity, may request special accommodations, and may need more time off. I have my own business, and disclosing my diagnosis is essential to my mission. But you should be very careful about doing so.

How to "come out":

There are many ways to come out. You can do so slowly and quietly or you can make it a celebration. Except for with my close friends, I hated the thought of coming out to people one by one and explaining what bipolar was, so I decided to come out to everyone else at once. Initially, I started a mental-health-related petition. I posted it on my Facebook page and encouraged people to sign it. The petition included a short bio of myself and why I started the petition, including my mental health condition. In the Facebook post, I also included a link to Diana Ross's "I'm Coming Out" classic. About five years later, I came out more formerly with a video of my recovery. I was overwhelmed by the touching and encouraging feedback I received. Several people posted very supportive comments. Not one single person on my Facebook page said anything at all negative. It made me very happy, surprised me, and greatly comforted me.

How much to disclose

You don't have to disclose every single detail of your experience. Disclose only what you're comfortable disclosing, and don't be afraid to tell people that you don't feel like talking about it in more detail. Reliving past experiences can be triggering for some people. Many people don't know others who are "out" about their mental health condition, so they may be curious about your experiences. When they ask about your condition, they are not necessarily trying to pry or intentionally trying to make you feel uncomfortable.

Special considerations

Coming out with mental health conditions requires you to be thick-skinned. You may be subject to more stigma, and you may develop higher sensitivity to stigma in the short term. People in your life may treat you differently. They may also gossip about you. People may exclude you from social gatherings. They may also feel awkward about what to say to you. Mental health is a difficult topic for many people. Some people may pity you.

Your immediate family may get upset with you for being so open about your condition. Unfortunately, stigma impacts not only people with mental health struggles but also their supporters. Even worse, your immediate family may have stigmatizing views toward you as well. Your parents may fear that they may be judged by others and be accused of being bad parents.

Importantly, once you're out . . . you're out. You can't take it back. You may regret the decision for some time. So make sure you carefully consider it and are prepared. Even more importantly, always be proud of who you are.

Over time, your coming out should cause friends, family, and others around you to see the realities and possibilities of mental health conditions. We hope, as so many of us know, that people realize that those of us with bipolar are no different than anyone else—that while bipolar may be part of us, it is not all of us. It's a serious condition, just like many others that many different people experience. People may admire you for your courage and bravery, the hope and inspiration you share with others. They will see the real you. Your example should serve as a powerful tool against stigma. Over time, people will have to refuse the common stigmas based on your courageous example.

Originally published in *bpHope*, Sept. 11, 2019.

11
The Example Celebrities with Mental Illness Set
Izzy Gonçalves

We have seen the story many times: a celebrity starts behaving erratically, and it's plastered across headlines. Their actions become increasingly self-destructive. People might question if it's an issue with drugs or alcohol. Their friends and family may express concern. The downward spiral continues. Then, the announcement - they've gone to rehab or a hospital to get help. In some cases, we learn the reason is bipolar disorder, depression, anxiety or another mental illness.

If that celebrity shares their diagnosis, it can be illuminating to people who follow them. In particular, people with mental illness might welcome a high-profile person coming out about their condition. They might feel less alone or even feel a sense of pride from what they have in common with a celebrity. They might feel better about themselves. Society might also revisit its perceptions and expectations of those with mental illness. The "celebrity endorsement" might help reduce stigma and shift public attitudes around mental illness.

But is the example set by that celebrity helpful? Being famous is often about creating and managing a public image. So, it's fair to question the authenticity and motives of their coming out. In fact, some celebrities romanticize aspects of mental illness, such as the connection between certain conditions and creativity. For example, Kanye West has openly disclosed that he has bipolar disorder. He has suggested that it enhances his creativity and artistry, and even suggests that it is a "superpower" in his lyrics.

The Good and the Bad

It is clear that mental illness "celebrity endorsements" are not all the same. While the mental health community would hope that celebrities only raise awareness in a positive way, it is possible that their behaviors perpetuate stigma. The celebrity's message may not be the most informed or helpful.

Sometimes, a celebrity discusses their refusal or reluctance to take medication. They make it sound like they don't need medication or that it stifles their creativity. This can be a particularly risky message. Medication is critical for so many, particularly those with severe mental illness. Celebrities may be accomplished and admired, but they are not doctors.

However, some celebrities speak very frankly about their diagnosis and struggles. They focus more on the challenges they encounter. One example is Saturday Night Live cast member Pete Davidson. A couple of years ago, he disclosed that he has borderline personality disorder. His ups and downs have been very much on public display, particularly following his split from fiancée Ariana Grande last year. Pete has openly addressed his issues on and off the show. His story is a very relatable account of a young adult recently diagnosed and coping with mental illness, free of romanticism.

I believe that these celebrity examples can be very positive if they are authentic, not just a tool to raise celebrity status. If the celebrity is authentic in their ownership of mental illness, they should feel a sense of responsibility as a representative of this community.

For me, both the examples of Kanye West and Pete Davidson can be constructive but for different reasons. We can also pick and choose the parts of their message and story that are most relevant and sensible to us. For example, Kanye West's lyrics might offer valuable inspiration and empowerment to those struggling with mental illness. To consider my mental illness a superpower can be uplifting, but I might also need my medication to help control these powers. Pete Davidson's down-to-earth attitude can certainly increase understanding about mental illness. When celebrities share their meltdowns and challenges, their followers can relate and feel less alone. There is power in this empathy, a sense of shared experience and community.

If a celebrity is being honest about their mental health issues, their example is likely to be helpful. More of these "endorsements" can certainly help reduce stigma. This can help people with mental health issues avoid isolation and seek out treatment and support. It can help them find hope and inspiration to persist on their journey of recovery. These very visible examples of celebrities living with a mental illness also show that we are not alone. Mental illness does not discriminate. The rich and famous have it too.

Originally published in *National Alliance on Mental Illness Blog*, May 15, 2019.

Part III.
Treatment and Recovery

12
Finding the Best Psychiatrist for You
Katherine Ponte

I've had three psychiatrists over the last 12 years. A social worker referred me to the first while I was hospitalized. My spouse selected the second using a "top doctor" guide. These two psychiatrists had excellent credentials. I stayed with each for five years, but my condition did not improve with either. I was reluctant to find a new one. I had shared many years of intimate and difficult details of my life with each, and I didn't want to do it again. They assured me that they cared for me and were looking after my best interests.

Eventually, I reached a breaking point with my second psychiatrist. She refused to change my medication regimen, which was causing me to sleep 14 hours a day. I impulsively decided I was going to find a new psychiatrist that would allow me to live again.

Through this process, I realized searching for the best psychiatrist requires incredible care, research and consideration. You should spend as much time finding one as you would buying a house or a car. Finally finding that third psychiatrist, the right one for me, has been essential to my recovery.

Below are some of the steps you can take to find the right psychiatrist for you.

Step 1: Search

I started by seeing who is out there and compiling a list of potential doctors.

Asking for a Recommendation

Talking to any friends or family who also live with mental illness can be a great place to start. You can also ask your therapist or primary care doctor for a recommendation.

Searching Online Directories

There are several online directories for psychiatrists, but you should keep in mind that some only require a fee to be listed. A few directories include:

American Psychiatric Association, Psychopharmacologist Guide, U.S. News & World Report, Castle Connolly, Vitals, Health Grades, and Psychology Today. Geriatric Psychiatrists.

Checking Medical Centers

Medical centers are often affiliated with medical schools. Check the best medical schools first in the U.S. News & World Report. One example is Massachusetts General Hospital-Psychiatry, which is affiliated with Harvard Medical School. These doctors work for the hospital, but often have a private practice as well.

Looking for Subspecialties

This is where I really started my search and spent the most time. I wanted someone with a subspecialty in bipolar disorder, including medication management. Doctors with subspecialties often treat more difficult cases; they have more specialized knowledge in a narrow area such as addiction psychiatrists. The specialties often have their own organization. Websites for these organizations, such as the American Academy of Addiction Psychiatrist, may provide tools to help find a specialist.

Reading Medical Journals

There was no directory for the bipolar specialty, so I researched reputable academic journals for authors who had written about bipolar. I researched PubMed and spent countless hours scanning publication titles, skimming relevant articles and assembling a list of names from my research. I was able to put together a lengthy list of doctors. I then googled each name to try to locate an email address for them. I emailed at least 50 doctors. I sent them each a very brief email as follows:

"I have been living with bipolar disorder for over 15 years and have experienced no improvement in my condition to date. If possible, I would be very grateful for a referral to a psychiatrist that specializes in bipolar disorder in the New York Area."

These inquiries led me to two bipolar specialty clinics, which led me to my current, wonderful psychiatrist.

Step 2: Screen

Once you've identified a doctor or multiple doctors, you still have to screen them. The following are some important items to review:

- Insurance: Do they take your insurance?

- Education: Where did they complete medical school, residency, post-residency?

- Specialty board certifications: Do they have certifications related to your condition, such as psychopharmacology?

- Areas of expertise: How relevant is their expertise to you? Do you want a generalist or someone with expertise in a subspecialty?

- Academic affiliation: Do they teach psychiatry? If so, they may be more familiar with scientific research.

- Publications: Have they published any articles in peer reviewed journals or books, or produced any videos?

- Years of experience: Are you comfortable with their level of experience?

- Website: Does the description of their practice seem like a good fit for you?

- Search: Do they have any disciplinary actions or other issues that concern you?

Step 3: Consult

During your initial consultation try to assess the doctor's fit and practice style. You should try to make a list of questions and bring a list of current medications, any testing records, health records, and hospitalization records to the consultation.

I wanted a doctor that practiced shared-decision making - one willing to consider my life goals, answer my questions, address my concerns, provide options and help me pursue the best course of action. I wanted to fully participate in my care unlike my previous psychiatric experiences.

My psychiatrist was not conveniently located (a 3-hour round trip), but over time we found that virtual consultations worked well. He was also out-of-network for my insurance, so it was more costly than other options. However, I thought that the best care I could afford was worth the inconvenience and expense.

I understand that not everyone is able to afford out-of-network care. So, if your insurance does not provide adequate coverage for you to see your preferred psychiatrist regularly, a one-time consultation with them might be doables. Then, take their recommended treatment plan to a general psychiatrist or even your primary care physician.

It took a lot of research and time to find my doctor, but it was well worth it. Now I know I'm receiving the best care possible. He has helped me live a full and meaningful life since 2016. My only regret is that I didn't conduct a thorough search sooner. We all deserve the best care possible. And while it's out there, we may have to work hard to find it.

References

American Psychiatric Association: https://www.psychiatry.org
Psychopharmacologist Guide: https://ascpp.org
U.S. News & World Report: https://health.usnews.com/doctors/specialists-index
Castle Connolly: https://www.castleconnolly.com
Vitals: https://vitals.com
Health Grades: https://www.healthgrades.com
Psychology Today: https://www.psychologytoday.com/us
Geriatric Psychiatrists: https://www.aagponline.org
American Academy of Addiction Psychiatry: https://www.aaap.org
PubMed: https://pubmed.ncbi.nlm.nih.gov

Originally published in *National Alliance on Mental Illness Blog*, Apr. 8, 2020.

13
Hope Starts with Mutual Peer Support
Katherine Ponte

Stigma says things will only get worse, that you'll never get better, have a job, a family, or happiness. But it doesn't need to be this way. With peer and family support, the right health care providers, and allies, you can reach recovery. After a 15-year struggle with severe bipolar I disorder with psychosis, it happened to me. It started with peer support, which renewed my hope.

Peer support works. There is strong evidence that it works. And it is just plain common sense that it should help. But peer support is too often an underappreciated and underutilized resource. Mutual peer support offers what other relationships typically cannot because peers share similar experiences and relatable perspectives. We can inspire hope and help guide each other. We model recovery and can motivate each other towards it. This type of bond increases the empathy we feel towards each other. We are there for each other, for small and big victories, setbacks and disappointments. It's reciprocal. We receive and give help; care and are cared for; empower and self-empower; and learn and teach coping strategies, self-care approaches, and insights. Together we make each other stronger and better prepared for the challenges we face each and every day, even once we reach recovery.

Recovery is not a destination. There is no cure for serious mental illness. It is a journey we'll be on for the rest of our lives, and we need peer support to sustain and help guide us.

The mere knowledge that I had peers pulled me out of isolation and withdrawal. Once I connected, interacting with peers made me get out of the house. I had lost many friends during the times I was most ill due to a lack of understanding, empathy, and compassion. Peers offered me friendship when I was without. They made me feel wanted and needed. With peers I found myself in a stigma- and discrimination-free environment.

My mental illness was and is a small part of me, but when I was highly symptomatic I let it define me. I found others that felt like me, and together we began to realize that we were so much more than our mental illness. We are like anyone else living with a health challenge, including people living with other serious chronic conditions. In each other, we found ourselves, a larger community of people with similar challenges. We can bring out the best in each other. We are not afraid to be who we are, mental illness and all. We don't have to pretend to be well. We don't have to be afraid that we'll lose those friendships and relationships because of our mental illness. We are part of a community of empathy and compassion. This is stigma's kryptonite.

Having hope in place, you want stability, to work harder to achieve it. Stability can allow us to dream again of the life goals we thought we had lost to our mental illness, that which we never thought would again be possible. Mental illness takes away our hope that those dreams might come true, but it doesn't take away our need, our desire to dream and pursue our dreams.

But too many people get stuck in a stability that targets mere symptom control and nothing more. They don't allow themselves to dream. Their view of the possible stops at stability. Having exposure to enough peers can show the true reaches of possibility. Symptom control is not enough. We want and need recovery. Symptom control did not make me want to get up out of bed in the morning. I was happy to be stable, but so much more is possible. But it requires work. It requires self-determination – to take ownership of your illness and outcomes.

I demanded and insisted that life goals be the target of my treatment, and shared decision-making was my treatment model of choice. I did not stop until I found a doctor willing to treat me as I deserved to be treated. I knew that I needed one willing to believe that I could and should achieve my dreams, even with my mental illness. My mental illness might have influenced my dreams, but that doesn't mean my dreams had to be less ambitious. Each of us must have our own life goals, which must be of our own choosing, to truly achieve fulfillment in life.

I was blessed to have peer-inspired hope, loving family support, and exceptional medical care to reach recovery. The right combination allowed me to reach recovery in just three short years. After fifteen long years without hope, five severe manic episodes one leading to arrest), psychosis, suicidal depression, and three involuntary hospitalizations, I've now been relatively symptom free for three years. My recovery journey will continue to evolve for the rest of my life, but it's on a really good, hopeful path, one I can build on.

Now, I have much improved family relationships, I have a job that I love, helping others just like me. So many people with mental illness want to return to the old life, before they got sick, their former selves. I don't want to. I have never been happier in my life. Having mental illness one gains a deeper appreciation of what life should be all about. Mental illness may take a lot away from us, but the struggle can ultimately help bring us closer to understanding the meaning of our lives.

People always ask me how I got here. It's within all of us. We just need a "little" help bringing it out. That "little" help is often peer support. We all deserve and are worthy of recovery. We have to help each other to achieve it. We have to work together to achieve it as a community. That "little" help can have enormous outcomes. It's the power of hope unlocking the need to dream again.

That's what peer support is all about. My hope started and continues to be inspired by my peers, and that's what it can do for so many people living with mental illness. I hope all people with mental illness can experience what I did, because this community needs more recovery. The hardest part about peer support is sometimes finding our peers.

Fountain House is an exemplary model of a community of peers, which has benefited so many and could benefit so many more. The world needs a "little more" Fountain House in how society treats people with mental illness. I hope it continues to inspire Clubhouses around the world. Because we peers have a lot of hope to share and we need each other.

Originally published in *Fountain House Blog*, Jun. 25, 2019.

14

The Effectiveness of Peer Support within the Context of Mental Illness

Professor Larry Davidson, Ph.D.,
School of Medicine, Yale University

Impact of peer support on recipients of peer support

Emerging evidence suggests that peer support delivered through multiple modalities (e.g., face-to-face, group based, online, etc.) has a positive impact on a range of outcomes among persons with varying types of mental illness. One early narrative review showed that peer staff functioned at least as well as non-peer staff and that peers who were engaged in traditional mental health roles (e.g., as case managers, etc.) facilitated similar or better outcomes among recipients of care relative to non-peers in those same roles (Davidson et al., 2012). Since that time, peer staff have increasingly been trained and hired to perform more unique peer-based roles (i.e., roles that explicitly incorporate and build on their lived experiences of recovery), and improvements have been found in numerous domains.

One meta-analysis of randomized controlled trials evaluating peer support delivered to persons with severe mental illnesses (e.g., schizophrenia, bipolar disorder, etc.), for example, revealed that peer support had a positive impact on recovery, empowerment, and hope (Lloyd-Evans et al., 2014). A second systematic review of multiple methodologies (e.g., randomized controlled trials, cross-sectional studies, etc.) evaluating different types of peer support delivered to persons with serious mental illnesses revealed that such support led to higher levels of engagement with care and patient activation for self-care; lower levels of inpatient service use; and better relationships with service providers (Chinman et al., 2014). A third systematic review of randomized controlled trials, randomized trials, and pre-post trials examining the impact of online peer support for youth with different mental illnesses (e.g., eating disorders, depression, anxiety, etc.) found that some peer-delivered interventions reduced anxiety, depression, and amount of time smoking tobacco (Ali et al., 2015). Finally, a recent narrative review found that being supported by peer staff contributed to increases in hope, empowerment, and quality of life (Bellamy et al., 2017).

In addition to these quantitative reviews, emerging qualitative evidence also highlights the importance and effectiveness of peer support. A recent meta-synthesis of qualitative studies on this topic revealed that recipients of peer support viewed peer support workers as important role models for recovery. They felt peer support workers fostered hope and motivation, and led to increases in their social network size. Recipients of peer support felt they could more easily connect with peer support workers relative to traditional mental health workers and that peer support workers possessed "lay" knowledge (i.e., "street smarts") that they found useful (Walker & Bryant, 2013).

Impact of peer support on providers of peer support

In addition to benefiting recipients of peer support, providers of peer support may also benefit from carrying out their work. For example, one pioneering qualitative study revealed how providing peer support fostered greater awareness and understanding about one's own mental illness; increased self-care; improved symptoms and overall sense of stability; greater positive emotions; improved self-concept and awareness of one's own personal strengths; and a greater self-acceptance and sense of empowerment. Through providing peer support, providers adopted new life perspectives; identified new meaning in the experiences they had; and improved their relationships with others (Moran et al., 2011).

A more recent quantitative study evaluating perceptions of peer support across the state of Pennsylvania revealed that working as a peer support worker was associated with reductions in traditional mental health service use (e.g., hospital visits); and that this work helped peer support workers develop new applicable life skills and feel more hopeful for the future. Being a peer support worker also provided opportunities to contribute to their employers and "give back" (Salzer et al., 2013). Similarly, a study of peer support workers across the United States revealed that peer support workers identified helping others and supporting their own recovery as the most rewarding aspects of their jobs (Cronise et al., 2016).

The effectiveness of peer support within the context physical illnesses

In addition to having a positive impact among persons with mental illnesses, receiving peer support may benefit persons experiencing physical illnesses.

53

Impact of peer support among persons with cancer

One systematic review of multiple study types identified several randomized controlled trials that demonstrated benefits of peer support for cancer. These included increases in self-efficacy and confidence and lower levels of depression, stress, and post-traumatic stress symptoms (Hoey et al., 2008). One qualitative study evaluating nine peer support groups for cancer across Australia revealed that peer support fostered a sense of community among support group members that was often difficult to experience outside the group. The peer support group setting facilitated honesty, empathy, acceptance and openness among group members, and provided a safe space for people to express their emotions and vulnerabilities. The group also distilled practical, day-to-day knowledge. Recipients of peer support also reflected on how taboo subjects such as death could be more easily discussed within the support group compared to with family or friends, who would often just encourage them to adopt a positive attitude in the face of their diagnosis. Finally, group members described experiencing positive changes after attending the group, namely, by becoming more open, humorous, confident, patient and tolerant (Ussher et al., 2006).

Impact of peer support on persons with diabetes and heart disease

Peer support may also yield some benefits for persons with diabetes. Specifically, one meta-analysis revealed that peer support interventions were associated with improvements in systolic blood pressure, but not with other cardiovascular disease risk factors (Patil et al., 2018). In persons with heart disease, one meta-analysis revealed that peer support increased self-efficacy and activity; reduced pain; and led to fewer visits to the emergency room (Parry & Watt-Watson, 2010).

Impact of peer support on positive and negative health behaviors

In addition to supporting persons experiencing physical illnesses, peer support initiatives have been implemented to improve or promote healthy behavior. For instance, one systematic review and meta-analysis revealed that peer support can improve breastfeeding practices among mothers. Specifically, the review revealed that peer support improved exclusive breastfeeding duration, particularly among mothers in lower middle income countries; facilitated breastfeeding initiation within a child's first hour of life; and reduced prelacteal feeding (Shakya et al., 2017).

Finally, in addition to encouraging adaptive health behavior, peer support may also reduce maladaptive heath behaviors. A recent systematic review and meta-analysis revealed that peer support interventions lowered the odds of smoking, drinking alcohol, and smoking cannabis relative to persons in control conditions (MacArthur et al., 2016).

Larry Davidson, Ph.D. is a Professor of Psychiatry and Director of the Program for Recovery and Community Health at the School of Medicine, Yale University. He is the author and co-author of over 450 publications on the processes of recovery from and in serious mental illnesses and addictions and the development and evaluation of innovative policies and programs to promote the recovery and community inclusion of individuals with these conditions.

References

Ali, K., Farrer, L., Gulliver, A., & Griffiths, K. M. (2015). Online Peer-to-Peer Support for Young People With Mental Health Problems: A Systematic Review. *JMIR Mental Health, 2*(2), e19. doi:10.2196/mental.4418.
Bellamy, C., Schmutte, T., & Davidson, L. (2017). An update on the growing evidence base for peer support. *Mental Health and Social Inclusion, 21*(3), 161-167.
Cronise, R., Teixeira, C., Rogers, E. S., & Harrington, S. (2016). The peer support workforce: Results of a national survey. *Psychiatric Rehabilitation Journal, 39*(3), 211.
Davidson, L., Bellamy, C., Guy, K., & Miller, R. (2012). Peer support among persons with severe mental illnesses: a review of evidence and experience. *World psychiatry official journal of the World Psychiatric Association (WPA), 11*(2), 123-128.
Hoey, L. M., Ieropoli, S. C., White, V. M., & Jefford, M. (2008). Systematic review of peer-support programs for people with cancer. *Patient Education and Counseling, 70*(3), 315-337.
Lloyd-Evans, B., Mayo-Wilson, E., Harrison, B., Istead, H., Brown, E., Pilling, S., et al. (2014). A systematic review and meta-analysis of randomised controlled trials of peer support for people with severe mental illness. *BMC Psychiatry, 14*(1), 39. doi:10.1186/1471-244x-14-39.
MacArthur, G. J., Harrison, S., Caldwell, D. M., Hickman, M., & Campbell, R. (2016). Peer-led interventions to prevent tobacco, alcohol and/or drug use among young people aged 11–21 years: a systematic review and meta-analysis. *Addiction, 111*(3), 391-407.
Matthew Chinman, Ph.D., Preethy George, Ph.D., Richard H. Dougherty, Ph.D.,

55

Allen S. Daniels, Ed.D., Sushmita Shoma Ghose, Ph.D., Anita Swift, M.S.W., and, et al. (2014). Peer Support Services for Individuals With Serious Mental Illnesses: Assessing the Evidence. *Psychiatric Services, 65*(4), 429-441. doi:10.1176/appi.ps.201300244.

Moran, G. S., Russinova, Z., Gidugu, V., Yim, J. Y., & Sprague, C. (2011). Benefits and Mechanisms of Recovery Among Peer Providers With Psychiatric Illnesses. *Qualitative Health Research, 22*(3), 304-319. doi:10.1177/1049732311420578.

Parry, M., & Watt-Watson, J. (2010). Peer Support Intervention Trials for Individuals with Heart Disease: A Systematic Review. *European Journal of Cardiovascular Nursing, 9*(1), 57-67. doi:10.1016/j.ejcnurse.2009.10.002.

Patil, S. J., Ruppar, T., Koopman, R. J., Lindbloom, E. J., Elliott, S. G., Mehr, D. R., et al. (2018). Effect of peer support interventions on cardiovascular disease risk factors in adults with diabetes: a systematic review and meta-analysis. *BMC public health, 18*(1), 398.

Salzer, M. S., Darr, N., Calhoun, G., Boyer, W., Loss, R. E., Goessel, J., et al. (2013). Benefits of working as a certified peer specialist: Results from a statewide survey. *Psychiatric Rehabilitation Journal, 36*(3), 219.

Shakya, P., Kunieda, M. K., Koyama, M., Rai, S. S., Miyaguchi, M., Dhakal, S., et al. (2017). Effectiveness of community-based peer support for mothers to improve their breastfeeding practices: A systematic review and meta-analysis. *PloS one, 12*(5), e0177434.

Ussher, J., Kirsten, L., Butow, P., & Sandoval, M. (2006). What do cancer support groups provide which other supportive relationships do not? The experience of peer support groups for people with cancer. *Social science & medicine, 62*(10), 2565-2576.

Walker, G., & Bryant, W. (2013). Peer support in adult mental health services: A metasynthesis of qualitative findings. *Psychiatric Rehabilitation Journal, 36*(1), 28.

Originally published in *ForLikeMinds Evidence*, 2019.

15
Family-to-Family Peer Support
Professor Larry Davidson, Ph.D.,
School of Medicine, Yale University

Family members often play a key role in supporting their loved ones throughout their recovery from mental and physical illnesses. As such, family members may have several support needs, many of which may be addressed through family-to-family peer support. Through family peer support, family members who care for loved ones with varying illnesses receive support from other family members who also have cared, or care, for ill relatives. Several forms of family peer support exist; for instance, such support may delivered by a provider to multiple families meeting together in a group, through mutual support groups, online or phone support, and individual family consultations. The effectiveness and impact of this type of peer support has been evaluated in several studies across different health contexts.

Family peer support for emerging mental health challenges

Several studies have investigated the impact or effectiveness of family peer support within the context of an emerging mental health challenge. For instance, one qualitative study examining the impact of family peer support on parents caring for children with behavioral difficulties revealed that peer support led to them to experience improved family relationships and happier families; become more empathic and accepting of others; develop greater confidence and knowledge; experience a sense of achievement; and see possibilities for new opportunities, including ways of helping other parents (Thomson, Michelson, & Day, 2015).

Other studies conducted within the context of emerging psychotic disorders have also revealed benefits of family peer support. One quantitative study (Levasseur, Ferrari, McIlwaine, & Iyer, 2018) exploring the impact of a family-run peer support group identified several benefits of peer support. These included developing greater knowledge about psychosis and its treatment; increased knowledge on how to cope with psychosis; and learning strategies to better care for themselves and their loved ones. In addition, families felt the support group provided emotional support. A qualitative study (Petrakis, Bloom, & Oxley, 2014) aimed at evaluating a family-run peer support intervention for families identified similar benefits. Importantly, family members reported the intervention helped them feel less lonely; express feelings and be listened to; experience a sense of cohesion with the group; develop greater knowledge about mental illness; experience reductions in stigma and shame; and develop better strategies for supporting their loves one.

Family peer support in the context of established mental health challenges

- Family peer support may also benefit careers whose loved ones are past the emerging stages of mental illnesses. In the context of psychotic disorders, one systematic review of all the quantitative and qualitative studies on family-to-family peer support (Chien & Norman, 2009) found that such support increased knowledge about psychosis, how it is treated, and how to access services; helped reduce caregiver burden and distress; and increased family members' social support, sense of cohesion with peer support group members, and their own ability to cope with stress.

- A series of studies examining family-to-family peer support in the context of mental illnesses more broadly also identified benefits of peer support. For instance, a pilot study examining the impact of a family peer support intervention (NAMI Family-to-Family Education Program) revealed that over time, family members felt greater empowerment within their communities, with their families, and within the mental healthcare system; and also experienced less worry and displeasure about their loved ones (Dixon, 2001). A follow-up study of this intervention also showed that peer support led to improved knowledge, empowerment, and family members' self-care strategies (Dixon et al., 2004). A third evaluation of this intervention revealed that it increased family members' sense of empowerment within their own families, communities and health service systems; increased their knowledge of mental illness; improved their acceptance of mental illness and problem solving techniques; and reduced their levels of anxiety and depression (Dixon et al., 2011).

- A series of studies evaluating the Journey of Hope intervention comparing family members who received family peer support to a control group revealed that family peer support improved satisfaction with caregiving and decreased need for information about caregiving (Pickett-Schenk, Bennett, et al., 2006). The intervention also decreased depressive symptoms and led to enhancements in emotional role functioning, greater vitality, and better relationships with their loved ones (Pickett-Schenk, Cook, et al., 2006). Finally, the intervention increased knowledge about ways to cope with their loved one's illness (Pickett-Schenk, Lippincott, Bennett, & Steigman, 2008).

- While most studies have focused on family peer support received or provided by adult caregivers, one study suggests that youth living with parents or siblings with mental illnesses may also benefit from family-based peer support (Foster, Lewis, & McCloughen, 2014). Specifically, results of a qualitative study revealed that through engaging in a peer support program, youth developed new relationships with peers and other staff at the program; acquired new roles as peer mentors; fostered a sense of belonging and experienced less loneliness; developed greater confidence, strength, courage, and higher self-appraisals; felt less blame about, and became more accepting of, their parents' mental health challenges; and found ways to give back to others and foster well-being in other people.

Family peer support for neurodevelopmental and physical illnesses

In addition to the evidence showing the benefits for family-to-family peer support within the context of mental health challenges, several studies have revealed the benefits of family peer support for families whose loved ones have neurodevelopmental or physical health challenges. For instance, a recent study used interviews and questionnaires to investigate the impact of a family peer support intervention for parents of children with a range of complex needs (e.g., Fragile X, congenital muscular dystrophy, Microcephaly, genetic disorders, Autism Spectrum Disorders, etc.) from the perspectives of both providers and recipients of this intervention (Bray, Carter, Sanders, Blake, & Keegan, 2017). Benefits that providers of the intervention identified included gaining a sense of purpose and accomplishment; developing new skills and prospects for the future; feeling less isolated, burdened, and more hopeful for the future; as well as experiencing improved mental well-being. Benefits that recipients of the intervention identified included feeling inspired, more confident, hopeful, and feeling less alone, burdened and distressed. Echoing these findings, results from a randomized controlled trial of family peer support for parents of children diagnosed with an Autism Spectrum Disorder revealed that parents who received peer support experienced less distress relative to parents who did not; and families who received peer support showed increased knowledge about Autism following the trial at a level comparable to families who did not (Bray et al., 2017).

Larry Davidson, Ph.D. is a Professor of Psychiatry and Director of the Program for Recovery and Community Health at the School of Medicine, Yale University. He is the author and co-author of over 450 publications on the processes of recovery from and in serious mental illnesses and addictions and the development and evaluation of innovative policies and programs to promote the recovery and community inclusion of individuals with these conditions.

References

Bray, L., Carter, B., Sanders, C., et al. (2017). Parent-to-parent peer support for parents of children with a disability: A mixed method study. Patient Education and Counseling, 100(8), 1537-1543. doi:10.1016/j.pec.2017.03.004.

Chien, W. T., & Norman, I. (2009). The effectiveness and active ingredients of mutual support groups for family caregivers of people with psychotic disorders: a literature review. International Journal of Nursing Studies, 46(12), 1604-1623. doi:10.1016/j.ijnurstu.2009.04.003.

Dixon, L., Lucksted, A., Stewart, B., et al. (2004). Outcomes of the peer-taught 12-week family-to-family education program for severe mental illness. Acta Psychiatrica Scandinavica, 109(3), 207-215.

Dixon L, S. B., Burland J, Delahanty J, et al. (2001). Pilot Study of the Effectiveness of the Family-to-Family Education Program. Psychiatric Services, 52(7), 965-967. doi:10.1176/appi.ps.52.7.965.

Dixon, L. B., Lucksted, A., Medoff, D. R., et al. (2011). Outcomes of a randomized study of a peer-taught Family-to-Family Education Program for mental illness. Psychiatr Services, 62(6), 591-597. doi:10.1176/ps.62.6.pss6206_0591.

Foster, K., Lewis, P., & McCloughen, A. (2014). Experiences of peer support for children and adolescents whose parents and siblings have mental illness. Journal of Child and Adolescent Psychiatric Nursing, 27(2), 61-67. doi:10.1111/jcap.12072.

Levasseur, M. A., Ferrari, M., McIlwaine, S., et. Al. (2018). Peer-driven family support services in the context of first-episode psychosis: Participant perceptions from a Canadian early intervention programme. Early Intervention in Psychiatry. doi:10.1111/eip.12771.

Petrakis, M., Bloom, H., & Oxley, J. (2014). Family Perceptions of Benefits and Barriers to First Episode Psychosis Carer Group Participation AU - Social Work in Mental Health, 12(2), 99-116. doi:10.1080/15332985.2013.836587.

Pickett-Schenk, S. A., Bennett, C., Cook, J. A., et al. (2006). Changes in caregiving satisfaction and information needs among relatives of adults with mental illness: results of a randomized evaluation of a family-led education intervention. American Journal of Orthopsychiatry, 76(4), 545-553. doi:10.1037/0002-9432.76.4.545.

Pickett-Schenk, S. A., Cook, J. A., Steigman, P., et al. (2006). Psychological well-being and relationship outcomes in a randomized study of family-led education. Archives of General Psychiatry, 63(9), 1043-1050. doi:10.1001/archpsyc.63.9.1043.

Pickett-Schenk, S. A., Lippincott, R. C., Bennett, C., et al. (2008). Improving knowledge about mental illness through family-led education: the journey of hope. Psychiatric Services, 59(1), 49-56. doi:10.1176/ps.2008.59.1.49.

Thomson, S., Michelson, D., & Day, C. (2015). From parent to 'peer facilitator': a qualitative study of a peer-led parenting programme. Child: Care, Health and Development, 41(1), 76-83. doi:10.1111/cch.12132.

Originally published in *ForLikeMinds Evidence,* 2019.

16
Shared Decision-making:
Getting a Say in Your Care
Katherine Ponte

I felt very stigmatized by my former psychiatrist. I often felt alienated, belittled, disempowered and invalidated. I felt unable to meaningfully contribute to my care, much less have a say. This significantly weakened both my comfort with her and my treatment outcomes.

In sharp contrast, my current psychiatrist's approach of shared decision-making encourages me to take greater ownership of my care and treatment. Shared decision-making is when a person and their mental health care provider collaborate to create a treatment plan. The patient's responsibility is to let the doctor know their goals and concerns for treatment. The health care provider's job is to provide expert advice about options. Then together, they discuss the risks, benefits and expectations of alternatives.

Having this different relationship dynamic with my doctor has significantly improved both my symptoms and my life.

The Benefits of Shared Decision-making

Here are a few differences between the care I received from my former psychiatrist and my current psychiatrist that show the potential benefits of shared decision-making for different treatment goals.

Goal: I want to be fully functioning and have a career.

Former psychiatrist: I felt that she cared little about my goals beyond stability. She characterized my career aspirations as a delusion of grandiosity. She offered me little alternatives to my medication regimen. She only focused on treating my symptoms, which left me in a state of almost constant sedation. My situation had not improved over five years of treatment. Our relationship became combative at times, and I questioned if her medical advice would allow me to achieve my goals. It was very discouraging, and I felt disempowered.

Current psychiatrist: My doctor did not question my goals—he respected them. He gave me options that would help me and asked me to decide on the appropriate course of action. I felt compelled to be both fully compliant and follow his guidance and advice, which I had complete confidence in. I felt validated and empowered. In just over a year of treatment with him, I had achieved my three main treatment goals.

Sleep

Goal: I do not want to live a life where I sleep 14 hours a day due to medication.

Former psychiatrist: Whenever I questioned the medication regimen, she dismissed my concerns by pointing to the degrees on her wall. When I was sleeping 14 hours a day, she told me I was in the best state she'd ever seen me. She told me I was stable. I agreed with her, but it was because I couldn't stay awake. It was difficult to imagine the possibility of recovery, but I felt that my life didn't have to be this way.

Current psychiatrist: He reduced the dose of the medication that was causing me so much sedation and suggested I try a stimulant. It was not a conservative approach for someone with bipolar disorder, but he said that there was research to support doing this, and he would monitor me very closely. He felt it might be worth the risk, which could be managed and eliminated if it produced adverse effects. After one week of treatment with him, my sleep time was reduced from 14 to 10 hours a night.

Weight

Goal: I wanted to lose weight because as a side effect I gained 60 pounds in two months on one medication.

Former psychiatrist: She didn't seem to appreciate the huge impact such a rapid weight gain had on my self-esteem and well-being. She only changed my medication regimen after I threatened to stop taking it on my own. I was furious that she wasn't more understanding of my concerns. I was ready to risk my safety to come off the medication. I became and stayed obese during my treatment with her.

Current psychiatrist: He carefully explained to me why I was not losing weight. He reduced the dose of the medication that was making it difficult for me to lose weight. As he made the dosage adjustments, he closely monitored its effects on me. I was so relieved to hear that my medication regimen could be changed responsibly. After about a year with my new doctor, I was able to lose over 70 pounds. My self-esteem improved, and I was able to step out of my sweats and buy new clothes for the first time in two years. It felt like a huge accomplishment that previously wasn't attainable.

Inclusion

Goal: I don't want my doctor consulting my spouse on my treatment decisions without my knowledge or approval.

Former psychiatrist: She frequently communicated with my spouse directly. I was often not informed of the content or manner of communication. It often caught me by surprise and made me feel angry and excluded. I felt that she listened more to my spouse than me. I actually wanted my treatment to fail out of spite, to show her that she didn't know what was best for me. I also lost trust in my spouse. I hid my symptoms from him when I was struggling out of fear he might "snitch" on me to my psychiatrist. My condition significantly deteriorated and even led to one of my hospitalizations.

Current psychiatrist: My new doctor listens to concerns raised by my spouse in a form we have all agreed to. He does not adjust my treatment without speaking and consulting with me first. The communication style between the three of us works really well and has led to a significant improvement in my relationship with my spouse. I have even allowed my spouse to take a bigger role in my care.

Feeling alienated from one's own care can pose a great obstacle for people with mental illness to reach recovery. It felt like my old psychiatrist questioned my capacity to achieve a fulfilling life and therefore acted as a barrier to reaching my goals. I would have reached recovery much sooner had I been treated using a shared decision-making approach all along.

People need to realize the important role they have in defining what's best for them, with the help of expert guidance. It is your life after all.

Originally published in *National Alliance on Mental Illness Blog*, Apr. 17, 2020.

17
Families Can Work Together
Izzy Gonçalves

Part I

Over 15 years, my spouse and I struggled with her seve
disorder. We went through weeks-long psychiatric hospitalizations, disrupted relationships and stalled personal and professional goals. Eventually, I took grudging ownership of her treatment. We resented each other, and we didn't work together.

I now know that the most effective treatment requires the person with the mental illness, their doctors and their supporters to work together. Frankly, through much of my spouse's illness, I thought I knew better, and her doctor at the time reinforced it. Her doctor and I communicated directly and largely controlled her treatment. She became less secure in her treatment as her doctor and I became a team.

As she started to find strength and hope from peer support, she wanted to take more control. So, she took a stand. She changed doctors and forced me to adjust my role in her treatment. I was furious. I saw that she was at high risk of another manic episode as she tried to make this change. However, things actually worked out.

We entered a recovery phase that I didn't know was possible. It wasn't the smoothest transition, but we became partners in her treatment. I discovered that things could be better, that we could both live fuller lives. That we could have more control over the condition's uncertainties.

With this new mindset, we both decided to get organized about her treatment and recovery. We did this by using a Collaborative Care Plan (CCP) (see Appendix I. Additional Resources). Using the CCP, a family team works together to develop treatment goals, responsibilities and action plans to facilitate recovery.

As we reflect on our experience, we recognize that reaching recovery would have been easier if we had been working more closely together all along. A CCP could have helped open up the communication and cooperation between us earlier. It would have helped us address practical issues and challenges created by my spouse's illness.

Treatment Team Guiding Principles

The three parties in collaborative care are the person with the condition (the "individual"), their family or other loved ones, and the clinician(s). The individual is often the most reluctant to participate in the plan, reinforcing the need for particular focus on their interests and perspective. The CCP seeks to maximize the individual's engagement with the collaborative care process. Based on our experience, the guiding principles of the CCP are:

- Individuals, family members and clinicians are a team.

- Care is individual-driven while the family and clinician play critical supporting roles.

- Treatment should be recovery- and wellness-oriented and should emphasize the individual's strengths.

- Evidence-based and emerging best practices should guide treatment decisions.

- Clinicians should provide individuals and family members ongoing guidance and skills training, especially crisis management, enabling them to better manage the illness.

- The treatment team should use a structured, but flexible, problem-solving approach to address issues and break them down into small, manageable steps.

- The team should acknowledge and address the possibility of impaired capacity *before* an emergency, including the potential need for involuntary treatment.

Strategies for Effective Communication

Communication across the treatment team is key to developing and implementing a CCP. Individuals, families and clinicians must have mutual respect for each other's experiences, preferences and goals. Each party should feel that their feelings and opinions matter. Such a setting allows for open discussion and problem-solving.

With that in mind, it's important to be very deliberate and attentive to communication. The following strategies may help improve

66

communication.

Listen to Each Other. There is no communication without listening. Here are a few strategies to help better communication through listening:

- Active Listening

- Reflective Listening

- Reframing

- Motivational Interviewing

Write Thoughts Down Before Saying Them. An effective strategy is for each participant to write down their views as specific questions are addressed. This allows for sharing and comparing everyone's views while also providing time to think about how to word statements in a respectful and non-triggering way.

Avoid Judgment. An individual may construe judgmental statements as authoritative and controlling, which will hinder communication. Judgmental statements are often difficult to avoid, particularly in intimate family settings, and may come out spontaneously in conversation. It helps to be particularly aware of the potential impact of statements to loved ones with mental illness.

Approaching potentially concerning behaviors with empathy and understanding may help address the behavior objectively without being judgmental. For example, instead of pressing an adult child to find a job, the parent might offer to help with the job search.

Preparing for the Uncertainties of Mental Illness

Recovery is not synonymous with "cured." People in recovery must work to remain in recovery and be prepared to address future periods of instability. Key components of the plan will include responsibilities for addressing triggers and early warning signs, mental health crises and even incapacitation (loss of function).

For example, with my years of experience supporting and caring for my spouse, I have become highly attuned to early warning signs of a potential manic episode. These include difficulty sleeping and religious preoccupation. As a part of developing our CCP, my spouse had to recognize my particular sensitivity to these indicators. My spouse had to agree to respect and validate my observations. In such cases, I have her approval to contact her doctor with my concerns as long as I tell her about my communication.

Another key component is conflict resolution. Many families grapple with when to hold their loved one accountable for troubling actions. Perhaps those actions were beyond their control, driven by their mental illness. Again, taking a deliberate and comprehensive approach is helpful. The individual and family member can each draw up a list of negative behaviors for discussion and place them into categories: accountable or beyond control.

The discussion will allow each party to point out items they think are missing or incorrectly categorized from the other's list. This list will also provide a basis for discussing and agreeing to a contingency plan for specific behaviors. This advanced planning will help take the uncertainty out of potential crisis situations. It also allows the individual to feel like they continue to have control.

Mental illness can seem impossible. But the fact is that communication and planning can allow us to problem-solve and prepare for the challenges that mental illness presents. A CCP can help organize our support team, improve communication and develop the strategies that make recovery from mental illness very possible.

Originally published in *National Alliance on Mental Illness Blog,* Nov. 4, 2019.

18
Finding the Best Medication Regimen
Katherine Ponte

After I received my diagnosis, I did not want to take my psychiatric medications. I thought the illness was just a phase and would pass. I doubted that a pill could address my erratic behavior or take away my pain and suffering. I tried anyway, but I struggled for 10 years to find the right medication. The process was incredibly frustrating and discouraging.

Eventually, I found a wonderful doctor. He showed me that medication could help me live the life I wanted, even with bipolar. Together, we found the best medication regimen for me, and I was able to get on the path to recovery. My mother recently sent a card to my doctor with a message: "Thank you for giving us our Kathy back."

Through this process, I learned a lot about medication. I would like to share some of this information, so other mothers, like mine, can feel that their children are getting the best possible care.

Finding the Right Health Care Provider

A primary care doctor, psychiatrist or psychiatric nurse practitioner may prescribe medication. A psychopharmacologist, who is a psychiatrist with expertise in medication management and more experience treating serious mental illness, can also prescribe medication.

Finding a good psychiatrist, or any other mental health provider, requires careful research. The most important factor to consider is if they fit what you are looking for, which can be critical to good outcomes.

It's advisable to carefully question your health care provider about medications so that you know what to expect, including activity and lifestyle restrictions and possible interactions with other medications. The most common questions are: What are my options? How long will it take to be effective? What are the possible side effects? What if it doesn't work? No question is too small, and doctors should encourage their patients to ask them.

Treatment should be person-centered and individualized. It can help to use a shared decision-making approach (SDM). Under SDM, a doctor will provide recommendations based on their expertise and ask the patient for their preference. It can be a very empowering approach and increase adherence. Treatment should offer hope by focusing on the pursuit of life goals rather than merely treating symptoms and avoiding risks.

Person-centered care and shared decision-making made me willing to try an entirely new medication regimen. I found a new psychiatrist who better fit my goals, which bolstered my confidence and my commitment to treatment.

Adhering to Your Prescription

Over 60% of people with serious mental illness do not take their psychiatric medication as prescribed. Partial or complete nonadherence to psychiatric medications is associated with many adverse outcomes. These include "exacerbation and relapse of symptoms, impaired functioning, suicidal behavior, increased hospitalizations and emergency room use and increased health care costs."

Those who agree to try medication may become nonadherent for many reasons, but adverse side effects are usually the primary reason. This happened to me. One medication caused me to gain 60 pounds in two months and another had me sleeping 14 hours a day. In both cases, trying to get off these medications led to an episode and hospitalization. I also once stopped taking medication because I believed I was "cured" when I started feeling better.

I also feared medication shaming, which is not uncommon for psychotropic medication. In fact, it is so prevalent that one of SNL's cast members, Pete Davidson, who lives with borderline personality disorder, addressed it on a show segment stating: "There's no shame in the medicine game. I'm on'em. It's great."

Family and friends may also negatively influence a person's decision to take medication if they tell the person that they do not need medication. It's no surprise that the greater the difference between consumer and caregiver attitudes towards taking medication, the greater the risk of nonadherence.

There are many ways to encourage adherence. In my case, medication was key, and it was critical for me believe that it could help me achieve my life goals. Stability was not enough for me. I wanted recovery, my doctor and family to be responsive to my concerns, and side effects to be minimal.

A few other ways to promote adherence to prescription medicates:

- Therapy

- Community health workers and peer support

- Financial incentives

- Electronic medication measurement

- Pharmacy-based reminders, such as those that send notifications to health care providers when a patient does not refill a prescription on time

Ultimately, taking medication requires weighing the pros and cons with a doctor. But once you have committed to trying medication, adhering to your doctor's prescription is key — even if people, including loved ones, tell you that you don't need it.

Integrating Holistic Care

An integrated treatment approach that addresses medical, psychiatric and social aspects can be highly beneficial. Research shows that medication with therapy is the most effective approach. The examples of others living well with mental illness on medication can also be incredibly powerful.

A caregiver can be a helpful part of the treatment plan. Their input and observations about the loved one's condition and progress can be valuable to the doctor. This approach often includes a Collaborative Care Plan (see Appendix I. Additional Resources).

An integrated approach can be helpful for people living with a co-occurring disorder (e.g., mental illness and substance use) or comorbidity (a mental illness and physical condition). Additional treatment providers may be required to effectively address all conditions. Failing to adequately address one condition may make it difficult to address the other condition(s).

Remembering that Patience is Key

Medications may not work quickly, and many people give up too soon.

Often, finding the right medication is an exercise of trial and error by the doctor to achieve a regimen that is most effective while minimizing adverse effects. This process can be long and discouraging.

I understand how that feels. I've been there. I don't like taking medications, or that my medications serve as a daily reminder that I have mental illness. But I need them to survive. I owe it to myself and my loved ones to take good care of myself. And you do too.

We may experience many setbacks, disappointments and mistakes along the way to find our best medication regimen, but we can't give up. We must view every trial and error as a learning experience to bring us closer and closer to recovery.

References

Medications Frequently Asked Questions: https://bit.ly/3e4IDbV
What to Expect From Your Medications: https://bit.ly/2zTH15I
Recommendations for Providers on Person-Centered Approaches to Assess and Improve Medication Adherence: https://bit.ly/3bImjTT

Originally published in National Alliance on Mental Illness Blog, Mar. 30, 2020.

19

A Risk Too Big Not to Take: A Story of Recovery
Katherine Ponte

Six hundred milligrams of quetiapine (Seroquel) a day—a doctor acquaintance would later tell me it was enough to take down a horse. Exaggeration or not, within 5 minutes of taking my nighttime medication, I couldn't keep from falling down and would sleep for over 12 hours straight. I was groggy all day. I was calm and controllable, but certainly not in control. My doctor viewed my behavior as evidence that I was well. And I understand that feeling groggy was better than the uncontrolled emotion and delusion of a full-blown manic episode. Feeling "comfortably numb" was the best I could expect. That Pink Floyd lyric took on even deeper personal meaning.

I was stable, but I didn't have much of a life. This once dynamic, vibrant lawyer and Wharton School M.B.A. graduate was now expected to resolve herself to nothing more than a sedated life. Forget prior career and family goals. They were all too much for me to achieve with this "handicap." How could I question my doctor's advice? Certainly, the number 1 priority was to prevent a future manic episode and hospitalization.

Despite the prescription-induced fog, I knew that I wanted a better life, as close to normal as possible. I understood the importance of respecting and treating my condition, yet I wanted to explore options for a more active and fulfilling life. I lobbied vigorously for a reduction in my quetiapine dose for months, but my doctor strongly resisted. It felt as though she had cast me into a zombie and would never lift the spell. As a result, I started experiencing suicidal depression. The choice I faced became clearer each day. It might have seemed risky, but doing nothing would have been a bigger risk.

I reached my epiphany in the wee hours of Sunday, April 10, 2016. I had been sleeping 14 hours a day for months, but for the past several days I couldn't sleep at all. I was hypomanic, teetering on manic. I was trying not to show it, but it was nearly impossible to hide. I had begun fighting with my husband, who started to sense pressure building toward a potential full manic eruption. He said that he couldn't deal with another "episode." All weekend I had been exchanging emails with my psychiatrist. I was anguished. I had been very unhappy with her treatment for a long time, but she was highly esteemed, had impeccable credentials, and was my spouse's trusted confidante about my treatment. Over 5 years, I had shared with her the most intimate and painful details of my life. Did I want to go through that again with someone new? Should I just settle with this existence? Could I even find anyone better?

That night I lay awake dreaming of a better life. Before dawn, I composed one more e-mail to my psychiatrist, this time terminating our relationship. In the past, these sorts of off-hour, pressured e-mails were a tell-tale sign for my family and friends that I was experiencing an episode of mania. I hesitated to send it for fear it would precipitate my hospitalization and its traumatizing physical and chemical restraints. But I knew that I had to make it clear that she was no longer my doctor. At 8:48 a.m., I summoned my courage and pressed the send button. Admittedly, the termination was medically unadvisable, and my husband was incensed. But I knew it was long overdue. Ultimately, it was lifesaving.

For the next 24 hours, I tried to stay as stable as possible. But remaining stable is extremely difficult when you have severe bipolar I disorder with psychosis and you've just been triggered. I had scheduled a consultation with another psychiatrist for the next day. He had agreed to see me, but not to treat me just yet.

In the preceding weeks, I had become increasingly consumed with finding a new doctor who might be able to treat my condition and allow me to live a full life. I spent countless hours researching on the Internet and firing off e-mail inquiries to find a top doctor. I hadn't found anyone I liked. I live in New York City, home to hundreds of psychiatrists, but it was an inquiry to a psychiatrist in California that led me to a referral in another state. I knew little of this psychiatrist, and I wasn't exactly in the best state of mind to make a careful and thoughtful assessment. In any event, I felt he was my only option. Although he had strong credentials, I was making a big leap to reject the care of my Manhattan-pedigreed doctor and restart with somebody new. Perhaps my hypomania was making me impulsive. Perhaps it was the fluttering of hope inside me, finally coming back to life after having lain dormant for so long. Early the next day, I was at Grand Central Station catching a train to the suburbs, followed by a cab to his office. I didn't know what to expect, but I hoped for the best.

I arrived early and anxious. He had no idea of all that had led up to that visit, and I didn't want to give any indication of this being anything more than a regular consultation. But I am certain he knew I was not well. Within 5 minutes, we got to the heart of the matter. I wanted to stop taking quetiapine and would be open to exploring alternatives. We met for about 2 hours. He respectfully listened to all my concerns and carefully reviewed and discussed each one. He mapped out my pharmaceutical options on a whiteboard. He carefully explained each one, and its pros and cons, asked me for my preference, and provided his recommendations—until that moment, I had never experienced shared decision making. I followed his advice.

Within 48 hours, I went from sleeping 14 hours a day to 10 hours, and in the coming months, I was down to 8 or 9 hours. I had captured an additional 4 hours of daily awake time. Imagine what you could do with an extra 4 hours a day? It was like being given more life. Within 3 months, the changes were far more than I could have even imagined. In that time, he identified my parathyroid disease, concluded that my treatment shouldn't prevent me from carrying a pregnancy, significantly reduced marital friction over my care, helped me lose over 50 pounds, helped me structure my days and be more productive, and all the while showed great care.

Above all, he nurtured my renewed hope for a fulfilling life. He guided me on my path to recovery and sustained me on my journey. I am now living my best life since I was first diagnosed over 15 years ago. Once he showed me that my illness could be treated and managed, I started to care more for myself so that I could achieve my potential. I began to envision a future that included not only bipolar disorder but also a life beyond it. Most importantly, I took more ownership of my condition and gained more control of my treatment. I began to work with a care team that includes a psychiatrist, a therapist, my spouse, and others.

I immersed myself in learning more about mental illness and recovery and began to recognize the benefits of peer support and sharing lived experience. Interacting with others with lived experience shows us that recovery is possible. It can reignite the hope dormant inside of us. So with the invaluable support of my spouse, I created ForLikeMinds, an online peer support community for people affected by mental illness. It allows members in similar circumstances to share their lived experience to rekindle hope, inspire, and inform each other's recovery journeys.

The odds of recovery may seem daunting for those of us who live silently with a diagnosis of mental illness. Finding the right medical treatment is critical. Each and every day we are at risk of becoming a sobering statistic, but good medical treatment can significantly improve these odds. People with serious mental illness have a significantly shorter average life expectancy. They are more likely to have a substance use condition, develop chronic disease, be arrested for crimes committed while ill, be unemployed, be dependent on government benefits, drop out of college, delay family planning, and have strained relationships with family. I myself had become a statistic many times over. Furthermore, of those who die from suicide, a great majority have a diagnosable mental disorder. The quantifiable costs to society of mental illness are in the trillions of dollars. Those statistics need not be so daunting. Those risks are too high and damaging to be accepted, without taking action.

Our lives are the result of risks both avoided and taken. Those of us with mental illness tend to focus on avoiding risks brought on by our condition. But the biggest risk of all is not to take the risk of recovery—resigning oneself to a life defined by mental illness instead of pursuing the possibilities of a fulfilling life. Each of us must accept this challenge. Acceptance is the act of ownership essential to reaching recovery. Others can support us, but they can't make us pursue recovery. The first act is to rekindle the hope that often lies long dormant within us. It is to believe that living with mental illness is living with possibility.

Originally published in *Psychiatric Services*, American Psychiatric Association, 11 Feb. 2020.

20
What Is Recovery?
Professor Larry Davidson, Ph.D.,
School of Medicine, Yale University

The onset of the kind of extreme emotional and social distress that can come to be defined as a "mental illness" can be traumatic and affect multiple areas of a person's life. Despite the suffering that such conditions may incur, people commonly recover. Multiple definitions of, and ways of conceptualizing, recovery following either an episode or prolonged period of mental illness exist. Two common definitions of recovery are clinical recovery and personal recovery.

Clinical recovery

Clinical recovery has often been conceptualized as a return to "normal" levels of functioning resembling how one was prior to the onset of a mental illness (Bellack, 2006). Persons are often considered in clinical recovery once they are no longer experiencing symptoms associated with a mental illness and are engaging in the occupational/educational and social activities they took part in before they became ill (Wunderink et al., 2009). About 38% of persons experiencing a mental illness such as psychosis experience full clinical recovery (Lally et al., 2017).

In addition, many people experience a resolution of symptoms of mental illness. About 58% of people experience full remission from positive symptoms (i.e., new perceptions or thoughts not shared by others) and negative symptoms (i.e., the absence or loss of emotions, thoughts and behaviors) following a first episode of psychosis (Lally et al., 2017). Individual studies have revealed an even higher proportion (68%) of people experience remission from positive symptoms alone (Jordan et al., 2018). A similarly high proportion of people (58%) may also return to prior functional roles following the onset of psychosis without experiencing remission from symptoms (Verma et al., 2012).

Personal recovery

In contrast with clinical recovery which has a single, precise definition, personal recovery has many definitions. One widely cited definition of personal recovery is that it is a "deeply personal, unique process of changing one's attitudes, values, feelings, goals, skills and/or roles. It is a way of living a satisfying, hopeful and contributing life even with the limitation caused by illness. Recovery involves the development of new meaning and purpose in one's life as one grows beyond the catastrophic effects of mental illness" (Anthony, 1993). Hence, personal recovery involves "recovering" a broader range of a person's sense of self and world compared to clinical recovery.

Davidson and colleagues (2005) identified common elements of personal recovery, which include renewing hope and commitment; redefining one's sense of self; coming to terms with and managing symptoms of the illness; being involved in meaningful activities; overcoming stigma; regaining control over one's life; being part of one's community; and exercising the same rights afforded to other citizens. In a systematic review and meta-synthesis, Leamy and colleagues identified five key processes of personal recovery, which include connectedness, hope and optimism for the future, identity, meaning in life and empowerment (Leamy et al., 2011). Based on the literature reviewed, they identified a recovery process that unfolds in five stages, which begins with pre-contemplation, and moves to the stages of contemplation, preparation, action, and growth and maintenance. Rates of personal recovery are high, with up to 54% experiencing personal recovery 20 years following the onset of psychosis (O'Keeffe et al., 2019).

Personal recovery may occur while a person is still experiencing symptoms of a mental illness; that is, even if they are not in clinical recovery. In such cases, personal recovery has been described as being in recovery with a mental illness. Personal recovery may also occur while persons are no longer affected by symptoms or signs of a mental illness (i.e., once they have experienced clinical recovery), also described as recovery from mental illness (Davidson & Roe, 2007). Hence, while clinical recovery and personal recovery may have separate definitions, they may still be inter-related phenomena, with a recent meta-analysis showing a small to moderate association between clinical and personal recovery from psychosis spectrum disorders (Van Eck et al., 2018).

What factors and processes are associated with recovery?

There are many paths to recovery: what may be important for one person's

78

recovery may not be important for another person's recovery. Despite such individual variation, some common facilitators and barriers to recovery have been identified across studies. People themselves play a very important role in their own recovery. However, relational, service-related, social and cultural factors also play key roles in both empowering and supporting persons with mental illnesses in their recovery.

Personal factors

People with mental illnesses play an active role in their own recovery. For instance, by acknowledging and accepting that one is in distress due to having anomalous or extreme experiences that others don't necessarily share and that can be understood to have to do with what health professionals would define as a "mental illness"; learning or figuring out ways to manage these challenging experiences, including using available treatments (e.g., medications and cognitive behavioral interventions), so that they do not interfere with living one's daily life; finding a sense of hope; finding the desire to change and grow; and fostering one's own sense of empowerment, self-control, and responsibility for one's overall life (Yung & Ensing, 1999).

Relational factors

Family members, significant others (e.g., spouses, etc.) and friends can help foster recovery by loving a person who is trying to recover from a mental illness; believing in their capacity to recover; allowing them to take risks; as well as by providing instrumental support (e.g., helping with finances, housing, etc.) and emotional support (e.g., listening to them, etc.) (Windell & Norman, 2013).

Mental health service-related factors

Mental health services can play an important role in supporting recovery from mental illnesses by fostering hope, empowerment, self-determination and agency; offering appropriate and non-coercive treatments that can reduce symptoms and promote functioning; and providing access to community-based resources and supports, including supported housing, employment, and education and peer support (Slade et al., 2014).

Social and cultural factors

Negative social attitudes and norms that stigmatize persons with mental illness are commonly described as barriers to recovery from mental illnesses (Wahl, 2012). In addition, insufficient funding of mental health services limits accessibility of mental health services and support resulting in unmet support needs (Pope et al., 2018; O'Keeffe et al., 2018). Conversely, many cultural practices, such as those tied to people's spiritual lives, may help facilitate recovery (Whitley, 2016).

Larry Davidson, Ph.D. is a Professor of Psychiatry and Director of the Program for Recovery and Community Health at the School of Medicine, Yale University. He is the author and co-author of over 450 publications on the processes of recovery from and in serious mental illnesses and addictions and the development and evaluation of innovative policies and programs to promote the recovery and community inclusion of individuals with these conditions.

References

Anthony, W. A. (1993). Recovery from mental illness: The guiding vision of the mental health service system in the 1990s. *Psychosocial Rehabilitation Journal*, 16(4), 11-23. doi:10.1037/h0095655.

Bellack, A. S. (2006). Scientific and consumer models of recovery in schizophrenia: concordance, contrasts, and implications. *Schizophrenia Bulletin*, 32(3), 432-442. doi:10.1093/schbul/sbj044.

Davidson, L., & Roe, D. (2007). Recovery from versus recovery in serious mental illness: One strategy for lessening confusion plaguing recovery. *Journal of Ment Health*, 16(4), 459-470. doi:10.1080/09638230701482394.

Jordan, G., Veru, F., Lepage, M., Joober, R., Malla, A., & Iyer, S. N. (2018). Pathways to functional outcomes following a first episode of psychosis: The roles of premorbid adjustment, verbal memory and symptom remission. *Australia and New Zealand Journal of Psychiatry*, 52(8), 793-803. doi:10.1177/0004867417747401.

Lally, J., Ajnakina, O., Stubbs, B., Cullinane, M., Murphy, K. C., Gaughran, F., et al. (2017). Remission and recovery from first-episode psychosis in adults: systematic review and meta-analysis of long-term outcome studies. *British Journal of Psychiatry*, 211(6), 350-358. doi:10.1192/bjp.bp.117.201475.

Leamy, M., Bird, V., Le Boutillier, C., Williams, J., & Slade, M. (2011). Conceptual framework for personal recovery in mental health: systematic review and narrative synthesis. *British Journal of Psychiatry*, 199(6), 445-452. doi:10.1192/bjp.bp.110.083733.

O'Keeffe, D., Hannigan, A., Doyle, R., Kinsella, A., Sheridan, A., Kelly, A., et al.

(2019). The iHOPE-20 study: Relationships between and prospective predictors of remission, clinical recovery, personal recovery and resilience 20 years on from a first episode psychosis. *Australia and New Zealand Journal of Psychiatry*, 4867419827648. doi:10.1177/0004867419827648.

O'Keeffe, D., Sheridan, A., Kelly, A., Doyle, R., Madigan, K., Lawlor, E., et al. (2018). 'Recovery' in the Real World: Service User Experiences of Mental Health Service Use and Recommendations for Change 20 Years on from a First Episode Psychosis. *Administration and Policy in Ment Health*, 45(4), 635-648. doi:10.1007/s10488-018 0851-4.

Pope, M. A., Jordan, G., Venkataraman, S., Malla, A. K., & Iyer, S. N. (2018). "Everyone Has a Role": *Perspectives of Service Users With First-Episode Psychosis, Family Caregivers, Treatment Providers, and Policymakers on Responsibility for Supporting Individuals With Mental Health Problems*. Qualative Health Research, 1049732318812422. doi:10.1177/1049732318812422.

Slade, M., Amering, M., Farkas, M., Hamilton, B., O'Hagan, M., Panther, G., et al. (2014). Uses and abuses of recovery: implementing recovery-oriented practices in mental health systems. *World Psychiatry*, 13(1), 12-20. doi:10.1002/wps.20084.

Van Eck, R. M., Burger, T. J., Vellinga, A., Schirmbeck, F., & de Haan, L. (2018). The Relationship Between Clinical and Personal Recovery in Patients With Schizophrenia Spectrum Disorders: A Systematic Review and Meta-analysis. *Schizophrenia Bulletin*, 44(3), 631-642. doi:10.1093/schbul/sbx088.

Verma, S., Subramaniam, M., Abdin, E., Poon, L.Y., Chong, S.A. (2012). Symptomatic and functional remission in patients with first-episode psychosis. *Acta Psychiatrica Scandinavica*, 124(4), 282-9. doi: 10.1111/j.1600-0447.2012.01883.

Wahl, O. F. (2012). Stigma as a barrier to recovery from mental illness. *Trends in Cognitive Science*, 16(1), 9-10. doi:10.1016/j.tics.2011.11.002.

Whitley, R. (2016). Ethno-Racial Variation in Recovery From Severe Mental Illness: A Qualitative Comparison. *The Canadian Journal of Psychiatry*, 61(6), 340-347. doi:10.1177/0706743716643740.

Windell, D., & Norman, R. M. (2013). A qualitative analysis of influences on recovery following a first episode of psychosis. *International Journal of Social Psychiatry*, 59(5), 493-500. doi:10.1177/0020764012443751.

Wunderink, L., Sytema, S., Nienhuis, F. J., & Wiersma, D. (2009). Clinical recovery in first-episode psychosis. *Schizophrenia Bulletin*, 35(2), 362-369. doi:10.1093/schbul/sbn143.

Yung, S. L., & Ensing, D. S. (1999). Exploring recovery from the perspective of people with psychiatric disabilities. *Psychiatric Rehabilitation Journal*, 22(3), 219-231.

Originally published in *ForLikeMinds Evidence*, 2019.

21
Psychiatric Rehabilitation
Professor Larry Davidson, Ph.D.,
School of Medicine, Yale University

Serious mental illnesses can affect functioning in many spheres of life, from disrupting school and work activities to impairing a person's ability to find and maintain affordable, quality housing (WHO, 2008). Resumption of employment, education, independent living, and functioning in other life domains has been shown to be important to recovery. While current treatments for mental illnesses, such as medications and psychotherapy, usually focus on reducing symptoms and distress, a number of other interventions are available which are designed specifically to assist people with mental illnesses to recover their degree of functioning in various life domains. These strategies fall under the broad category of "psychiatric rehabilitation." Briefly stated, psychiatric rehabilitation supports people in reclaiming meaningful, valued roles in the community and improving their quality of life (Corrigan & McCracken, 2005; Farkas & Anthony, 2010). Psychiatric rehabilitation is person-centered and embraces the central recovery values of self-determination, choice, and hope (Farkas & Anthony, 2010). In contrast to focusing on symptoms or illness, psychiatric rehabilitation focuses on helping individuals with mental illness develop the skills needed to function in the areas of importance to them (e.g., independent living, work/school, social activities) and providing environmental supports to facilitate their functioning (Anthony et al., 2002; Farkas & Anthony, 2010). These supports are usually provided in the community settings where these activities naturally take place, such as in one's home, work site, or classroom.

Established types of psychiatric rehabilitation include supported housing and employment / education, with increasing evidence accumulating for supported socialization / recreation and promise shown for supported spirituality. We review each below.

Supported employment and education

Mental illnesses typically emerge during a stage of life when individuals are completing school and entering the workforce or pursuing higher education (Killackey et al., 2006). As a result, work and school functioning is often disrupted. People with serious mental illnesses have much lower employment rates than the general population, with European estimates ranging from 10%-20% and American estimates from 3%-40% (Marwaha & Johnson, 2004). In addition to enabling financial independence, research has shown that employment is critical to recovery, providing a sense of meaning, pride, and self-esteem; helping cope with psychiatric disability; and improving quality of life, social functioning, satisfaction with leisure activities, and other indicators of recovery (Dunn et al., 2008; Charzynska et al., 2015). A large body of evidence supports the effectiveness of the Individual Placement and Support (IPS) model for helping persons with mental illness resume work or school (Killackey et al., 2008; Nuechterlein et al., 2008). The focus of supported employment and education is on helping individuals with mental illness quickly choose, get, and keep a job/course of study in real life work and school settings, while receiving skills training and support as needed (Corrigan & McCracken, 2005). Compared to those in "train and place" supported employment (in which individuals receive skills training first and are then placed in work or school settings), persons receiving IPS-style supported employment are more likely to obtain employment (and sooner), retain employment longer, spend more time employed, and earn more income, without increased hospitalization, symptoms, or disability (Frederick & VanderWeele, 2019; Corrigan & McCracken, 2005). Supported education has also been shown to be highly effective in improving academic engagement and success, without appearing to increase symptoms or relapse (Corrigan & McCracken, 2005).

Supported housing

People with serious mental illness often have difficulty maintaining affordable, quality housing, which in turn has a negative effect on their mental health. Indeed, independent living in quality housing is considered essential to recovery (Browne & Courtney, 2007). Supported housing has largely shifted from a "train and place" model, in which individuals with mental illness gradually progress from living in more structured, supervised settings to independent housing as they achieve independent living skills, to a "place and train" model (Corrigan & McCracken, 2005). This model, embodied by the Housing First (HF) approach, rapidly places individuals in independent housing of their choice and provides support and skills training as needed, without requiring that individuals first receive treatment or other interventions (Tabol et al., 2010). A recent study found that homeless or precariously housed adults with serious mental illness who received HF and assertive community treatment entered housing faster, remained stably housed longer, and experienced improved quality of life and community functioning compared to persons receiving treatment as usual (Aubry et al., 2015). In fact, persons receiving HF spent 71% of time in the preceding 24 months in stable housing while persons receiving usual care only spent 29% of time in stable housing. Persons in supported housing have also reported that exercising personal choice (e.g., socializing whenever and with whomever they want; choosing the decor and organization of their physical space) contributes to their recovery (Piat et al., 2019).

Supported socialization and recreation

Individuals with serious mental illness frequently experience a loss of social ties in the wake of the illness and have limited social networks and recreational activities (Davidson et al., 2004). Supported socialization and recreation are less well-established forms of psychiatric rehabilitation. However, in a randomized controlled trial of supported socialization in which individuals with mental illness were paired with a "consumer" or "non-consumer" volunteer partner (or no partner at all), supported socialization was associated with improved social functioning and self-esteem, though only for individuals who met with a non-consumer partner (Davidson et al., 2004). In another study, pairing community volunteers with persons with serious mental illness was found to increase social support and subjective well-being and decrease psychiatric symptoms after one year (McCorkle et al., 2008). A meta-analysis of befriending (i.e., deliberate friendship) also demonstrated that it was associated with improved quality of life (Siette et al., 2017).

Supported spirituality

Spirituality is an important component of recovery for many individuals with mental illness, leading some to propose that supported spirituality may be a promising avenue for psychiatric rehabilitation (Russinova & Blanch, 2007). Though not yet a mainstream practice, Fallot (2001) suggests that clinicians could use spirituality to support recovery for persons with mental illness by regularly exploring the nature and function of spiritual beliefs in a person's life via "spiritual assessments"; discussing spiritual and religious issues in group interventions; incorporating religion and spirituality into individual psychotherapy; and cultivating relationships with community resources providing religious and spiritual supports.

Conclusion

While these are the major areas of development in psychiatric rehabilitation, new advances are being made all of the time in promising new directions. People can be supported in pursuing almost any interest or activity they value—leading to such areas, for example, as supported pet ownership—being limited only by their imagination. This is encouraging, as a wealth of evidence suggests that psychiatric rehabilitation in its many forms can be a potent contributor to recovery.

For more information

Should you be interested in finding out about psychiatric rehabilitation programs or resources in your own community, and you are already participating in mental health care, ask your doctor, clinician, or other provider about possible referrals for these services. You can also contact your state's department of mental health or explore their website for available programs in your state. While these services may be provided by a diverse array of agencies, including clinics and hospitals, many rehabilitative services are provided by clubhouses and psychosocial rehabilitation centers where you may go for further information.

Larry Davidson, Ph.D. is a Professor of Psychiatry and Director of the Program for Recovery and Community Health at the School of Medicine, Yale University. He is the author and co-author of over 450 publications on the processes of recovery from and in serious mental illnesses and addictions and the development and evaluation of innovative policies and programs to promote the recovery and community inclusion of individuals with these conditions.

References

Anthony, W., Cohen, M., Farkas, M., et al. (2002). *Psychiatric Rehabilitation,* Second Edition. Center for Psychiatric Rehabilitation, Trustees of Boston University.

Aubry, T., Goering, P., Veldhuizen, S., et al. (2015). A multiple-city RCT of housing first with assertive community treatment for homeless Canadians with serious mental illness. *Psychiatric Services, 67*(3), 275-281.

Browne, G., & Courtney, M. (2007). Schizophrenia housing and supportive relationships. *International Journal of Mental Health Nursing, 16*(2), 73-80. doi:10.1111/j.1447-0349.2006.00447.x

Charzynska, K., Kucharska, K., & Mortimer, A. (2015). Does employment promote the process of recovery from schizophrenia? A review of the existing evidence. *International Journal of Occupational Medicine and Environmental Health, 28*(3), 407.

Corrigan, P. W., & McCracken, S. G. (2005). Place first, then train: An alternative to the medical model of psychiatric rehabilitation. *Social Work, 50*(1), 31-39.

Davidson, L., Shahar, G., Stayner, D. A., et al. (2004). Supported socialization for people with psychiatric disabilities: Lessons from a randomized controlled trial. *Journal of Community Psychology, 32*(4), 453-477.

Dunn, E. C., Wewiorski, N. J., & Rogers, E. S. (2008). The meaning and importance of employment to people in recovery from serious mental illness: results of a qualitative study. *Psychiatric Rehabilitation Journal, 32*(1), 59.

Fallot, R. D. (2001). Spirituality and religion in psychiatric rehabilitation and recovery from mental illness. *International Review of Psychiatry, 13*(2), 110-116.

Farkas, M., & Anthony, W. A. (2010). Psychiatric rehabilitation interventions: A review.
International Review of Psychiatry, 22(2), 114-129.

Frederick, D. E., & VanderWeele, T. J. (2019). Supported employment: Meta-analysis and review of randomized controlled trials of individual placement and support. *PloS One, 14*(2), e0212208.

Killackey, E. J., Jackson, H. J., Gleeson, J., et al. (2006). Exciting career opportunity beckons! Early intervention and vocational rehabilitation in first-episode psychosis: employing cautious optimism. *Australian and New Zealand Journal of Psychiatry, 40*, 951-962.

Killackey, E., Jackson, H. J., & McGorry, P. D. (2008). Vocational intervention in first-episode psychosis: individual placement and support v. treatment as usual. *The British Journal of Psychiatry, 193*(2), 114-120.

Marwaha, S., & Johnson, S. (2004). Schizophrenia and employment - a review. *Social Psychiatry and Psychiatric Epidemiology, 39*(5), 337-349. doi:10.1007/s00127-004-0762-4

McCorkle, B. H., Rogers, E. S., Dunn, et al. (2008). Increasing social support for individuals with serious mental illness: Evaluating the compeer model of intentional friendship. *Community Mental Health Journal, 44*(5), 359.

Nuechterlein, K. H., Subotnik, K. L., Turner, et al. (2008). Individual placement and support for individuals with recent-onset schizophrenia: integrating supported education and supported employment. *Psychiatric Rehabilitation Journal, 31*(4),

86

340-349.

Piat, M., Seida, K., & Padgett, D. (2019). Choice and personal recovery for people with serious mental illness living in supported housing. *Journal of Mental Health*, 1-8.

Siette, J., Cassidy, M., & Priebe, S. (2017). Effectiveness of befriending interventions: A systematic review and meta-analysis. *BMJ Open, 7*(4), e014304.

Tabol, C., Drebing, C., & Rosenheck, R. (2010). Studies of "supported" and "supportive" housing: A comprehensive review of model descriptions and measurement. *Evaluation and Program Planning, 33*(4), 446-456.

Russinova, Z., & Blanch, A. (2007). Supported spirituality: A new frontier in the recovery-oriented mental health system. *Psychiatric Rehabilitation Journal, 30*(4), 247-249.

World Health Organization. (2008). *The Global Burden of Disease: 2004 Update*. Geneva: Author.

Originally published in *ForLikeMinds Evidence*, 2019.

22
People with Mental Illness Can Work
Katherine Ponte

I was unemployed for many years while I was most ill. During that time, I felt worthless and dependent. Why? Because of the:

- debilitating impacts of mental illness.

- fear of having to explain my spotty resume due to multiple hospitalizations and depressive episodes.

- awareness that nothing I had done before I got sick seemed to count.

- prospect of having to start over.

- stigma that told me I could not work.

Stigma says to people with mental illness that we're not ambitious, motivated, intelligent or able. It says we're unable to handle stress, too sick and even potentially dangerous. However, these are all myths, and the common belief that people with mental illness cannot work is a myth.

Sadly, these misconceptions combined with a lack of support keeps many people with mental illness from working. According to survey data from 2010, "employment rates decreased with increasing mental illness severity", and "people with serious mental illness are less likely than people with no, mild or moderate mental illness to be employed after age 49."

This is a problem that needs our attention. People with mental illness can, should and often need to work.

The social costs of the unemployment and underemployment of people living with mental illness are incalculable: worsening health, additional health care costs, financial struggle for families, among many others.

Additionally, work gives a source of purpose and allows us to contribute to our families and society. Sustained employment is an incredibly important factor for recovery. And the majority of those with mental illness can succeed with appropriate support.

Programs that Support Employment

The existence of several employment support programs reflect that people like us are able to work and keep jobs. NAMI's Road to Recovery Report provides a good overview of these programs, which are all evidence-based. These include:

- American with Disabilities Act (ADA). Employers may be required under the ADA to provide reasonable accommodations, when requested, to an employee with a disability as long as it does not cause undue hardship on the employer. Examples include telecommuting, scheduling flexibility, sick leave, breaks and noise reduction.

- Many mental health workplace accommodations are low cost and easy to implement, but they can have a significant positive impact on both employees and employers. Accommodations that help people with disclosed mental illness might also help those with undisclosed mental illness feel more comfortable in the workplace. Additionally, it might encourage those that are not fully functioning in the workplace due to mental illness (presenteeism) to ask for accommodations as well. Presenteeism is very expensive to companies as it can cause significant productivity loss. And providing adequate accommodations to staff with disabilities has the potential to reduce those costs.

- Supported Employment – Individual Placement and Support (IPS). IPS programs seek to help people with mental illness choose, secure and keep competitive employment while providing ongoing individualized long-term support. They try to place people in jobs that match their talents and interests. IPS programs are highly effective. Competitive employment rates for individuals participating in IPS programs were close to 60% compared to 24% for individuals not in the programs. Yet, less than 2% of people served by state mental health systems received supported employment services.

- Assertive Community Treatment (ACT). ACT provides intensive support services to people with serious mental illness in the community. The program includes components such as individualized treatment, community integration and job placement. Each ACT team includes an employment specialist. All the different pieces of the program, including employment activities, are incorporated into the person's overall treatment plan.

- Clubhouses. Clubhouses are community-based centers open to individuals living with mental illness that offer supported employment programs. Members of Fountain House, the world's leading clubhouse for people living with serious mental illness, achieve an employment rate of 42% versus only 15% for people with serious mental illness in the general population.

- Some clubhouses also offer supported education programs. Supported education programs can help people living with mental illness enhance their job prospects. This is important as mental illness often onsets during prime academic years.

- The challenge of many hardships related to mental illness is not knowing what to do. In the case of getting people with mental illness back to work or school, we have evidence-based solutions. What we need is greater awareness of, investment in, and expansion of these programs.

People with Mental Illness Can Be Successful

Mental illness doesn't need to be an obstacle to employment. In fact, mental illness may be correlated with success in certain professions. For example, there are many successful entrepreneurs living with bipolar disorder. This makes sense as people with bipolar disorder are known to be highly creative and innovative. Also, entrepreneurs may have more flexibility around work hours and location which might better accommodate living with mental illness.

Another example is working in the health care sector. Lived experience can be invaluable when working in health care, particularly in mental health. We understand what it's like to live with mental illness and what it takes to reach recovery. Our perspective is different from that of clinicians and one that has proven to be highly beneficial as evidenced by the work of certified peer specialists (CPS).

CPSs are an emerging type of mental health care professional, a person with mental illness living in recovery who helps others reach recovery. They inspire hope by being a role model for recovery. They also build on their own confidence and empowerment through their sense of purpose and social connectedness. CPS work is considered a best practice by the Substance Abuse and Mental Health Services Administration and is Medicaid reimbursable in 39 states. Witnessing other peers in recovery inspired me to believe recovery was possible for me. This is why I proudly became a New York certified peer specialist-provisional.

In addition to working as a CPS, our lived experience can be extremely valuable and complementary to many mental health disciplines, including social work, therapy, psychology and psychiatry.

People with mental illness must be encouraged to enter or re-enter the workforce and offered reasonable support to do so. We must advocate for programs that support them getting jobs. We must hire them. And we must support businesses owned by them. These efforts benefit people living with mental illness, their families, workplaces and society. It benefits you and me. People with mental illness have so much to offer. Hopefully, one day we'll have equal opportunities to participate in the workforce.

References

NAMI's Road to Recovery Report: https://adobe.ly/2ygcvTg
American with Disabilities Act (ADA): https://bit.ly/2zcT0eS
Supported Employment: https://bit.ly/2ZeVdB8
Assertive Community Treatment (ACT): https://bit.ly/2zcVaes
Supported Education: https://bit.ly/3bFEEAU

Originally published in *National Alliance on Mental Illness Blog*, Oct. 21, 2019.

23
The Mental Health Movement in the Workplace
Katherine Ponte

The mental health movement in the workplace has been growing over the past several years. This focus is extremely important given the direct impact of work on mental health. The average person spends upwards of 40 hours a week working. Work is also a leading source of stress, which is a potential trigger of mental illness.

Companies have so much to gain from investing in their employees' mental health. Wellness increases productivity. Investing in employee wellness also increases company loyalty and improves recruitment.

If employees are more loyal and productive, often the company will be more successful. This positive feedback loop is benefits employers and employees. It's also beneficial to the mental health movement, where companies play an important role.

Companies have the power to influence their employees through mental health workplace policies, the public through marketing and mental health awareness campaigns their community through goodwill initiatives such as support for non-profits, and their competitors by making mental health benefits a competitive consideration in employee recruitment and retention.

How to Promote Mental Health in the Workplace

There are many actions companies can take to enhance workplace mental health.

Policies

Companies can implement clear policies and values supporting mental health.

Company leadership at all levels should:

- Foster a culture in which seeking help is a sign of strength.
- Reject and prohibit stigma.
- Encourage open and honest discussions with employees about

mental health issues, including anonymous feedback on workplace policies.

- Reinforce that "health" includes physical health and mental health.

- Recognize the spectrum of mental health conditions from emotional distress to diagnosable conditions, which requires access to different types of care.

- Dedicate company resources to supporting workplace mental health.

- Recognize that family challenges may impact mental health by developing policies to promote better work-life balance.

Recruitment

Companies can adopt recruiting practices that respect the potential contributions of candidates with mental illness, such as:

- Placing job announcements where people with mental illness are known to frequent, such as Clubhouses.

- Understanding that academic and work interruptions due to illness are common.

- Seeking to implement Supported Employment practices, which allow more people with mental health conditions to enter the workforce. This approach recognizes that the extremely high unemployment rates for people with mental illness are addressable.

- Supporting job market inclusion of more vulnerable mental health communities, including those with serious mental illness.

Accommodations

Employers should consider reasonable accommodations, such as those covered by the Americans with Disabilities Act. This flexibility may allow employees to work with more suitable work environments, schedules and time allowances for appointments.

Supervisor Trainings

Employers should train supervisors to identify emotional distress and implement strategies to assist employees who may be struggling. These strategies may include:

- Making employees more comfortable talking about mental health.

- Encouraging employees to seek mental health treatment when needed.

- Assuring employees that they will not be judged or disadvantaged for seeking treatment.

- Ensuring private and confidential discussions, which allows for building trust.

- Rewarding and praising an employee for proactively addressing mental health issues, including making use of workplace resources.

Education

Employers can require all employees to complete basic mental health education. This helps employees support colleagues facing challenges and self-identify areas of concern. These strategies may include:

- Using screening tools.

- Raising awareness of community resources.

- Providing teach-ins with therapists or other professionals, perhaps working with a mental health nonprofit to raise employee awareness and knowledge.

  o Train employees to better identify and manage certain work activities and environments that may trigger and exacerbate emotional distress. This can also include addressing coronavirus-specific triggers.

- Encouraging peer-to-peer engagement and support. Employers can also share online peer-based support communities, which can complement workplace initiatives.

Employee Benefits

An employer's benefits package is an important tool in promoting workplace mental health. Benefits packages with the following features may be particularly useful for promoting mental wealth:

- Good insurance coverage for mental health conditions, including a diverse and comprehensive range of mental health treatments and a range of in-network providers. Modalities covered should include hospitalization, 24-hour services, partial hospitalization, outpatient services, medical management, case management and psychological rehabilitation services.

- Employee Assistance Programs: Companies should offer and encourage employees to make use of these programs. They can help cope with day-to-day stresses and prevent them from growing into more significant health issues.

- Wellness Programs: Employers may offer on-site holistic wellness activities recognizing their positive impact on mental health. These programs might include meditation spaces, gym membership subsidies, mental health days, flex-time or peer-to-peer engagement.

- Remote Work: The coronavirus lock-down may show employers that telework is feasible as an ongoing option for employees. Employers can consider a ROWE model, which stands for Results Only Work Environment, whereby employees can work whenever and wherever they want as long as their work gets done. One study showed that ROWE promotes "employee wellness, particularly in terms of prevention behaviors."

External Support

Employers may support the work of mental health nonprofits and issues impacting the mental health community to further demonstrate company support for mental health. Notable initiatives could include:

- Matching for nonprofit donations.

- Promoting and organizing volunteer or service opportunities for employees

- Supporting parity for behavioral health coverage through direct and indirect advocacy.

- Helping disadvantaged communities, such as the incarcerated and homeless, where mental illness is most prevalent.

Corporate America does and *can* play a more impactful role in the mental health movement. Supporting people with emotional distress and mental health conditions supports *all* employees. It allows employees to work at their best and can significantly enhance corporate performance.

The growing and open discussion of mental health issues in society reinforces its importance to companies. Mental health initiatives are increasingly vital to corporate performance and corporate citizenship. They are a measure of the quality of a company. Good mental health is good business.

References

Workplace Strategies for Mental Health: https://bit.ly/2BFhb6J
American Psychiatric Association's Center for Workplace Mental Health: workplacementalhealth.org
One Mind at Work: onemind.org
Supported Employment: https://bit.ly/2AMu5Px
Accommodations: https://bit.ly/2zcT0eS

Originally published in *National Alliance on Mental Illness Blog*, Jun. 10, 2020.

24
Mental Health Peer Specialist Support
Professor Larry Davidson, Ph.D.,
School of Medicine, Yale University

What is it?

The concept of mental health peer support developed in the late 1980s and early 1990s as a product of the Mental Health Consumer/Survivor Advocacy Movement. After providing mutual support to each other for over two decades within the context of self-help groups and consumer run programs outside of the mental health service system, persons recovered or recovering from mental illnesses, who began to call themselves "peers," began to be formally trained and employed to provide similar kinds of support to other people struggling with mental health issues inside of the mental health system. At first, these services were similar to the roles already being played by paraprofessionals in mental health programs, such as case management and residential support, and these services were found to be equally effective when provided by such "peers" as when provided by non-peer paraprofessional staff (Davidson, Chinman, Kloos, et al., 1999).

Once the possibility of training and hiring peers was established, however, leaders in the peer movement began to identify and build on several aspects of the support that could be provided uniquely by persons with their own history of "lived experience" of recovery. These would be kinds of support, that is, that could only be provided by people who had "been there" themselves: people who had learned how to live with and recover from a serious mental illness wither on their own or who also had learned how to navigate both the social service and mental health service systems as part of their recovery. Having been in these shoes themselves earlier in their own lives, such peers could instill hope for recovery in others, could educate others about and provide role modeling in self-care, and could share their hard won knowledge, or "street smarts," about how to access and utilize the resources needed to build a safe, meaningful, and gratifying life in the community in the wake of a serious mental illness. As described below, such services have since been found to improve a range of outcomes among persons receiving these kinds of peer support.

Who offers it?

Mental health peer support can be provided by anyone who has lived with and recovered to some degree from a serious mental illness themselves, whether or not they did so with the help of formal mental health services. For these services to be paid for by Medicaid (the most common source of funding) or private insurance (less developed as a source of funding thus far), most states require the peers providing these services to have been formally trained and certified by an agency or program approved by the state for this purpose. While no formal, national records are kept at this time on the utilization of peer support, the Veterans Administration alone has trained and hired over 1,200 such peers and estimates of the number of peers hired across the U.S. are in the 10s of thousands. In addition to the U.S., large numbers of peers have been trained and deployed in similar ways throughout the English-speaking world (e.g., Canada, United Kingdom, Australia, and New Zealand) and across Western Europe, with peer support being in earlier stages in Asia, South America, and Africa (Stratford, Halpin, Phillips, et al., in press).

Where is it offered?

Initially, mental health peer support was offered through independent peer-run programs and through psychiatric rehabilitation programs and community mental health centers. In the mid 1990s, through the federal ACCESS program, peer staff were hired to conduct homeless outreach, with parallel developments in hiring peer staff on assertive community treatment teams. While less common in the U.S. thus far, peers have been hired through the National Health Service in England to staff psychiatric hospitals and inpatient units and, as mentioned above, all Veterans Administration medical centers have hired peer staff, who typically work in rehabilitative settings. At this point in time, it is possible to find peer staff working in practically every service setting across the continuum of care in some part of the U.S., with the majority working in outpatient, outreach, and rehabilitative programs.

Where else is peer support used?

What is now called peer support has been around in various forms since at least the late 18th century and in many different areas of life or health fields. The father of psychiatry, Phillipe Pinel, hired persons who had recovered from their own mental illnesses to staff is first mental hospital in Paris in the 1790s. The most well-know and perhaps ubiquitous form of peer support is the 12-step self-help group format that originated from Alcoholics Anonymous in the 1930s and which has since branched out into numerous groups for persons with other substance use and addictive disorders (e.g., Cocaine Anonymous, Gamblers Anonymous) as well as their family members (e.g., ALANON). Similarly, self-help groups and peer supports have been developed for persons with a variety of other health conditions (e.g., asthma, cancer) and life circumstances (e.g. loss of a spouse or child, divorce, or other traumatic events). While the leaders of such self-help groups are typically volunteers, rather than paid staff, many of these areas have also developed peer mentorship and outreach programs in which the support is provided by paid peers, similar to mental health peer support. Most recently, this has been seen as an important development within the context of the opioid epidemic, with "recovery coaches" being trained and hired to provide a range of outreach, mentorship, and other kinds of support to persons with substance use disorders.

What benefits have been attributed to peer support?

As mentioned above, peer staff were initially found to generate equal clinical outcomes to non-peer paraprofessional staff when functioning in conventional case management or residential support roles. Since the peer role has been more fully developed based on the unique contributions peers bring to this role given their life experiences and accumulated knowledge base, newer forms of peer support have been consistently shown to improve more recovery-oriented outcomes such as increases in hope, empowerment, self-care, and quality of life (Bellamy, Schmutte, & Davidson, 2017; Chinman, George, Dougherty, et al., 2014; Davidson, Bellamy, Guy, & Miller, 2012; Fuhr, Salisbury, De Silva, et al., 2014; Lloyd-Evans, Mayo-Wilson, Harrison, et al., 2014; Pitt, Lowe, Hill, et al., 2013). These outcomes are thought to be promoted through a combination of the following functions of peer support: combatting stigma and discrimination and instilling hope for recovery; role-modeling coping strategies and self-care skills; and sharing of the peer staff's accumulated life experiences with navigating the health and social service systems in order to engage the person in care and enable him or her to access available community resources.

What are the future prospects for peer support?

The two newest areas in which peer support has been developing are in providing on-line support through a combination of apps and telephone contact and in peers being trained and hired to provide health navigation services in addition to conventional peer support. Health navigation involves educating and supporting persons with mental illnesses in taking care of themselves and their health in the face of comorbid medical conditions such as diabetes and hypertension, which are common byproducts of the side effects of psychiatric medications, sedentary lifestyles, and a range of social determinants of health such as poverty, unstable housing, and prolonged unemployment to which persons with mental illnesses are also more likely to be susceptible. An initial systematic review of peer-delivered approaches to addressing the general health needs of persons with serious mental illnesses found health navigation and focusing on promoting self-care to hold the most promise (Cabassa, Camacho, Vélez-Grau, & Stefanic, 2017).

Larry Davidson, Ph.D. is a Professor of Psychiatry and Director of the Program for Recovery and Community Health at the School of Medicine, Yale University. He is the author and co-author of over 450 publications on the processes of recovery from and in serious mental illnesses and addictions and the development and evaluation of innovative policies and programs to promote the recovery and community inclusion of individuals with these conditions.

References

Bellamy, C., Schmutte, T., & Davidson, L. (2017). An update on the growing evidence base for peer support. Mental Health and Social Inclusion, 2017, 21(3), 161-167.

Cabassa, L.J., Camacho, D., Vélez-Grau, C.M., & Stefanic, A. (2017). Peer-based health interventions for people with serious mental illness: a systematic literature review. Journal of Psychiatric Research, 84, 80-9.

Chinman, M., George, P., Dougherty, R. H., Daniels, A. S., Ghose, S. S., Swift, A., & Delphin-Rittmon, M. E. (2014). Peer support services for individuals with serious mental illnesses: assessing the evidence. Psychiatric Services, 65(4), 429-41.

Davidson, L., Bellamy, C., Guy, K., & Miller, R. (2012). Peer support among persons with severe mental illnesses: a review of evidence and experience. World Psychiatry, 11(2), 123-128.

Davidson, L., Chinman, M., Kloos, B., Weingarten, R., Stayner, D., & Tebes, J.K. (1999). Peer support among individuals with severe mental illness: A review of the evidence. Clinical Psychology: Science and Practice, 1999, 6, 165-187.

Fuhr, D. C., Salisbury, T. T., De Silva, M. J., Atif, N., van Ginneken, N., Rahman, A., & Patel, V. (2014). Effectiveness of peer-delivered interventions for severe mental illness and depression on clinical and psychosocial outcomes: a systematic review and meta-analysis. Social Psychiatry and Psychiatric Epidemiology, 49(11), 1691-702.

Lloyd-Evans, B., Mayo-Wilson, E., Harrison, B., Istead, H., Brown, E., Pilling, S., . . . , Kendall, T. (2014). A systematic review and meta-analysis of randomised controlled trials of peer support for people with severe mental illness. BMC Psychiatry, 14(1), 39.

Pitt, V., Lowe, D., Hill, S., Prictor, M., Hetrick, S. E., Ryan, R., & Berends, L. (2013). Consumer-providers of care for adult clients of statutory mental health services. Cochrane Database Systematic Reviews. 3(9).

Stratford, A.C., Halpin, M., Phillips, K., Skerritt, F., Beales, A., Cheng, V., Hammond, M., O'Hagan, M., Loreto, C., Tiengtom, K., Kobe, B., Harrington, S., Fisher, D., & Davidson, L. (in press). The growth of peer support: An international charter. Journal of Mental Health.

Originally published in *ForLikeMinds Evidence*, 2019.

25
Building Mental Health Resilience
Katherine Ponte

Resilience is the process of finding healthy ways to adapt and cope with adversity and distress. Building resilience can be key to helping us get through the Coronavirus crisis and its aftermath. It can help protect us from various mental health conditions, such as depression, anxiety and traumatic stress. And it can help those of us who already have mental health conditions cope better.

Prior tragedies have shown the power of resilience. Knowing this, and how to build resilience, can be a source of great hope for many people. In fact, people can even experience emotional growth after a tragedy.

Building Resilience

Everybody's experience is different. Genetics can play a role, so certain resilience factors may come more naturally to some. Others may need to practice and build resilience skills. For those who are curious, the Connor-Davidson Resilience Scale assesses various dimensions associated with a person's resilience.

If you want to work towards being on the higher end of this scale, there are many evidence-based strategies to build resilience. These tactics have demonstrated positive impacts and may be helpful in addressing potential traumatic stress from the pandemic. The following strategies can contribute to resilience.

Practice Radical Acceptance

This pandemic is out of our control — we cannot will it away — and it is therefore important to *accept* the current situation for what it is. Being able to manage and cope with uncertainties we cannot control is a form of resilience. To practice this, you can apply Dialectical Behavioral Therapy's distress tolerance skills, particularly radical acceptance, to learn to be collected despite this crisis.

Embrace Realistic Optimism

This concept is the ability to identify challenges and overcome them by focusing on what is solvable. In the case of coronavirus, experts told us to expect steep increases in infections, but also that social distancing could "flatten the curve."

While it's important to understand the severity of the situation, it's even more important to focus on what we each can do to help lessen the negative impact, which in this case, is staying home as much as possible. Through realistic optimism, we can believe in our ability to flatten the curve and focus our efforts on making that a reality.

Also act on your sense of right or wrong. For example, respecting social distancing and not hoarding groceries safeguards us individually and collectively.

Reframe Negative Thoughts

Sometimes it's challenging to separate thoughts from feelings. Negative thoughts can be overwhelming and make you feel significantly worse. One way to overcome them is by reframing, or challenging, those negative thought patterns. Instead of telling yourself that "nothing will ever be the same," you can reframe it to "maybe something positive can come from this, such as employers allowing people to work from home more often."

Try Problem Solving

It can be helpful to address immediate concerns by thinking creatively. This approach can also help manage interruptions in daily routines. You may not be able to attend fitness classes anymore, but you can try online fitness classes. You may not be able to spend time with friends in person, but you can host a game night over Facetime or Zoom. You may not be able to go listen to live music, but you can tune-in to special programming, such as the Together at Home Concert.

Consider Adaptive Resilience

This concept is the ability to learn from the past, understand current capabilities and to anticipate tomorrow's threats. For example, the current crisis has increased awareness of issues in our health care system. You can engage in advocacy work to reform health care through nonprofits such as NAMI. Channeling your energy, or even distress, into trying to create positive change is a great example of resilience.

Find Resilience Role Models

Let yourself be inspired by the actions of historical and current heroes in the face of great adversity such as healthcare workers fighting the coronavirus. You can learn about them through movies, biographies or news stories. When you feel like you can't take this situation, or need a sense of strength, you can look to these role models and learn from them.

Be There for Others

Seek out and offer empathetic and compassionate support for friends, family and others in similar situations. It promotes understanding and coping for the person giving and receiving support.

You can also help people through mutual aid and other volunteer work. There are many ways to help high-risk groups, such as the elderly and other immune-suppressed or -compromised individuals in this crisis.

Find Humor When You Can

Humor is a powerful coping strategy. For example, it was extremely effective for Vietnam prisoners of war. Finding and sharing humor in aspects of this crisis (aka the great American Toilet Paper panic) can help us take control of our circumstances and connect with each other.

Practice Positivity

There are certain mindsets that can help build resilience: joy, gratitude, serenity, interest, hope, pride, amusement, inspiration, awe, and above all, love, which can occur in adverse circumstances. The Broaden-and-Build Theory states that positive thoughts and feelings broaden our awareness and encourage novel, varied and exploratory thoughts and actions, which help people build skills and resources. So, find what you are grateful for and write it down. Think about what gives you a sense of hope. And give love to those in your life.

Grow Beyond Resilience

In response to trauma, some people may experience tragic optimism. It's an ability to maintain hope and find meaning in life despite its inescapable pain, loss and suffering.

In addition to helping build resilience, these responses may culminate in posttraumatic growth (PTG). PTG is the experience of positive change that occurs as a result of the struggle with highly challenging life crises. It can manifest itself in many ways, including:

- Increased appreciation for life

- Strengthened relationships

- Boosted sense of personal strength

- Improved priorities

- Deepened existential and spiritual life

Now is a time to further reflect on the meaning and purpose of our lives. It can help us build resilience and grow beyond it. Achieving resilience and posttraumatic growth may take time, tremendous will power and determination — but it is possible.

Conclusion

During this difficult time, it is my sincerest hope that people will also look to the many examples of resilience in our mental illness community. No one knows the pain of isolation, loneliness, unemployment, debilitating illness and life-threatening circumstances like we do. Our condition may be chronic, but "still we rise."

The coronavirus and its aftermath will likely be the greatest challenge in recent memory, but we are all survivors. That is a large part of what defines humanity. We should never underestimate ourselves. Together, we will overcome the pandemic as individuals and as a society.

Further reading

Connor-Davidson Resilience Scale: https://bit.ly/3g76OYL
Post-Traumatic Growth Inventory: https://bit.ly/3cPxSd2
Dennis Charney, *Resilience: The Science of Mastering Life's Greatest Challenges*
Martin, Seligman, *Flourish: A Visionary New Understanding of Happiness and Well-Being*

Originally published in *National Alliance on Mental Illness Blog*, Apr. 20, 2020.

26
Ways to Manage and Cope with Stress
Katherine Ponte

My dad was dying. I hated my job. I was struggling with school. A classmate groped me in front of other classmates. I was having a nervous breakdown.

I wanted an explanation. I wanted something I could address to make me well. I wanted someone and something to blame. But all I was given was a label – bipolar disorder.

I might have been more willing to accept my diagnosis if someone had explained it to me in the context of the life events I was experiencing. It might have made sense to me if I had connected the diagnosis with those stressful events.

Many years later, I learned that my stressful life events did have something to do with how I was feeling, reacting and behaving. For people with a pre-existing genetic vulnerability to mental illness, severe levels of stress *can* trigger mental illness. Research has shown this connection for major depressive disorder (MDD), bipolar and schizophrenia.

High levels of stress can also cause an episode or make symptoms worse for someone who already has mental illness. For bipolar disorder, stress can contribute to hypomania and mania. For schizophrenia, it may contribute to hallucinations and delusions. And for MDD, it can deepen depression.

This is why managing stress is so important. In order to manage stress, we need to know the warning signs that stress levels are too high and learn healthy coping techniques.

Signs of Severe Stress

Not all stress is bad. In fact, it can be helpful for gaining motivation, building resilience and encouraging growth. However, stress can negatively affect a person and their health if not properly managed, especially for someone with mental illness.

The are many physical and emotional signs that stress is negatively affecting someone. In fact, according to the American Institute of Stress, there are 50 common signs and symptoms of too much stress.

One of the most common physical signs of high levels of stress is sleep deprivation. In one survey, over 40% of Americans reported that stress had prevented them from sleeping. Other physical signs include frequent headaches and aches and pains. Examples of emotional signs include anger, mood swings, difficultly concentrating and irritability.

Sources of Stress

Stress affects each person differently. A person's genes and prior experiences influence how sensitive they are to stressful life events. However, certain circumstances or life events are generally known to cause stress and can help pinpoint where an individual's symptoms might be coming from.

The Holmes-Rahe Stress Inventory scores a person's "stress inventory" using 43 stressful life events. Each event is assigned a numerical score. The higher the total score for all events, the more vulnerable a person is to a stress-induced health breakdown, which may include the triggering of mental illness.

The top three stressful life events identified by the inventory are the death of a spouse, divorce and marital separation. Illness is also a top stressful life event.

When stressful life events happen, we may not be able to change the situation or eliminate our stressors, but we can learn to manage our stress levels in a healthy way.

Methods for Managing Stress

There is no one size fits all strategy to managing stress – each person should identify which coping methods work best for them. It can help to develop coping strategies that address specific sources of stress. Also, the ability to easily incorporate coping strategies into your routine and lifestyle increases the likelihood of maintaining the practice. Keep in mind that small steps can have a big impact.

- Problem-focused coping - A person directly confronts a stressor or tries to find a solution to the stressor. For example, if having too many commitments is causing you stress, you may consider eliminating one of them to better manage the others. It can be tough to implement problem-focused coping if the sources are difficult to address, such as a stressful job situation or family relationship. In these cases, rather than grapple with the source of stress, an emotion-focused approach might be more effective.

- Emotion-focused coping - A person focuses on regulating their reaction to a stressor. This approach allows a person to accept their stressors and find ways to shift how they experience them. For example, if a family member causes you distress, you can journal your feelings or reframe your thoughts about the situation to better regulate your feelings.

- Wellness-focused coping - Encompasses a range of strategies that align with specific interests and sources of stress, or dimensions of wellness There are eight interdependent dimensions of wellness: physical, intellectual, financial, environmental, spiritual, social, occupational and emotional.

Physical: Any form of exercise can relieve stress. Research has found that 30% of adults felt less stressed after exercising.

Intellectual: Activities that engage your mind such as reading, journaling about emotions, and jigsaw puzzles are all helpful coping tools.

Financial: According to the American Psychological Association, money and finances are a top stressor for Americans. Money management resources can provide strategies and solutions for money-related stress.

Environmental: Spending time in nature and green spaces is shown to help relieve stress.

Spiritual: Connecting with yourself and the world around you through meditation, prayer, or other forms of spirituality can help provide meaning, comfort and stress relief.

Social: According to a 2015 survey, "43% of those who say they have no emotional support report that their overall stress has increased in the past year, compared to 26% of those who say they have emotional support." Staying in close touch with family and friends, seeking out opportunities to make new friends and participating in community activities are all useful methods for dealing with stress.

Occupational: Next to money, work is the second leading stressor with 60% of people finding work-related stress to be significant. One important form of occupational stress relief is to do work that you are truly passionate about, if possible. It's also helpful to take time to recharge and establish healthy boundaries and work/life balance.

Emotional: To address your emotional wellness, you can detach yourself from stressors, practice relaxation techniques, try reframing your thoughts, or go to therapy, among many other possibilities.

Stress is a persistent force in our lives. Many people have come to accept it as normal, even when it gets out of hand, and let it build. But changing our relationship with stress is critically important for improving our health and well-being.

Had I known that stress could trigger my bipolar, I would have done more to address the stressors in my life. We often hear "mental illness can happen to anyone." While this is true, we should also recognize that effectively managing stress can reduce the risk of developing mental illness or worsening symptoms. And this is one of the few tangible and actionable strategies we have to reduce that risk.

The goal is not to avoid stress but to manage it effectively. Stress is something we can and should address for the sake of our mental health.

References

Eight interdependent dimensions of wellness: https://adobe.ly/2WINf1s
A Wellness Approach: https://adobe.ly/3ga7GeK

Originally published in *National Alliance on Mental Illness Blog*, Jan. 13, 2020.

27
The Remarkable Human Animal Bond
Katherine Ponte

Why does the world over love Rin Tin Tin, Benji, Lassie, our furry babies? We find solace from daily pressures and sometimes human cruelties in cat videos and dog Instagram accounts. They soften our souls appealing to some purer loving part of ourselves. It's an inexplicable human animal bond, enduring friendships and emotional support, which many humans simply cannot find in other humans. They brighten so many people's lives with an estimated 67% of U.S. households (or 84.9 million homes) owning a pet. Nearly all pet owners consider pets to be members of their family. These bonds can be greater still between a person living with mental illness and their pet. In one study, 60% of people with chronic mental health conditions considered their pets to be as important as family members. The healing power of our little friends can be indescribable.

This was the case with my dearly departed cat Dude. Way back when I got him, I could have never imagined the critical, pure loving role that he would come to play in coping with my severe depression. He sensed it, he felt it, he lived it with me. He never left my side even when everyone else did, he never left me all alone, he rescued me many times in his instinctive caring way. I'd speak to him in the depths of my depression: "you love me, you'll always love me no matter what" and I'd hear his silent response.

These pets have a natural talent as support animals. They can play a valuable role in addressing mental health issues, as detailed below.

Benefits of the Human Animal Bond

Pet ownership has many possible mental health benefits. It has been shown to reduce stress, depression and anxiety and improve overall quality of life in many ways. Pets provide a calm presence, can divert negative thoughts, and promote exercise. Caring for pets can help commit owners to routines such as daily walking, create a sense of purpose and accomplishment, and facilitate social and community interactions and integration. Some of these benefits may be activated by merely petting or playing with pets. However, arguably the greatest direct benefit of pet ownership is emotional companionship. All loving pet owners know this, but the impact on people living with mental illness can be profound. It can be life-saving.

A literature review of people living with mental illness provides convincing evidence of this "pet effect". According to the literature review, which is consistent with my own personal experiences, pet ownership can reduce feelings of isolation and loneliness. Pets are an important, trusted and consistent source of unconditional love and affection. They intuitively provide this support in times of need and provide a distraction from ruminations on negative thoughts, including suicidal ideation. They are also valued as a "person" to speak to, because a person may speak to them without fear of judgment or the sense of being a burden. As they seemingly listen without response, there is no fear of interruptions, criticisms, and advice, and there is respect for boundaries and confidentiality. A pet is accepting of his/her owner without regard for their illness which may help normalize the owner's life. As a result, they make people feel good about themselves and provide reasons to live. For these reasons, some people prefer relationships with pets over humans, including family members.

Some of the negative aspects of pet ownership, include financial costs, housing concerns, obedience issues and distress that can result from the eventual loss of a pet.

Types of support animals

There are many types of support animals and interventions, The most common animal types are emotional support animals, service animals, and therapy animals.

Emotional support animals

Emotional support animals (ESAs) provide emotional support and comfort to their owners on a daily basis. Unlike service animals, they are not trained and do not perform specific tasks. ESAs can include dogs, cats, rabbits, birds, hamsters, horses and others. For your pet to be considered an ESA legally, you must have a prescription letter which is renewed yearly from a licensed therapist or doctor that states you have a mental disability and that an ESA is necessary for treatment. This is the only legal document governing ESAs. Note that many online companies sell fake

ESA certifications/registrations. ESAs are considered a reasonable accommodation under the Fair Housing Act (FHA), which allows tenants to reside with an ESA in a no-pet dwelling for no additional fee. Documentation may be required. Under the Air Carrier Access Act (ACAA), airlines must allow ESAs to accompany their handlers in the cabin of the aircraft at no cost subject to review of your prescription letter. Unusual animals such as snakes and rodents are not permitted to be ESAs. It may be possible to file an appeal where a landlord or carrier denies your request.

There is growing controversy over ESAs. Many people are suspected of misrepresenting pets as ESAs to obtain the privileges accorded to ESAs. The National Disability Rights Network has been a strong advocate in the area.

Service Dogs

A psychiatric service dog is defined as:

> "a dog that has been trained to perform tasks that assist individuals with disabilities to detect the onset of psychiatric episodes and lessen their effects. Tasks may include reminding the handler to take medicine, providing safety checks or room searches, or turning on lights for persons with Post Traumatic Stress Disorder ("PTSD"), interrupting self-mutilation by persons with dissociative identity disorders, and keeping disoriented individuals from danger."

Service animals are "working animals" and not pets. Only service animals, including dogs and miniature horses are accorded special privileges or considered a reasonable accommodation under the American with Disabilities Act (ADA) Services dogs are allowed in all public facilities even when a no pets policy exists and an employer may be required to allow a service dog in a place of employment to work alongside their handler. An employer may ask "If your dog is required because of a disability?" and "What work has your dog been trained to perform?" Service animals are entitled to the same rights as ESAs under the FHA and ACAA. Public facilities and employers may not require you to present documentation. You may register your dog with the U.S. Service Registry for free and voluntarily.

Service dogs have been shown to especially benefit veterans suffering from PTSD in many ways, including reduced PTSD symptoms and improved quality of life. They have also been shown to reduce anger and anxiety and enhance sleep. Specific tasks performed help veterans to cope with anxiety or panic attacks, and create space between the handler and other people. The best place to source a service dog is Assistance Dogs International, including Psychiatric Service Dog Partners. Training and costs of ownership can be prohibitive with some costing upwards of $20,000 for training alone. There are non-profits that provide veterans service dogs at no cost such as K9s for Warriors.

Therapy Animals

Trained therapy animals are typically certified dogs that accompany handlers in visits to hospitals, including psychiatric units, nursing homes and others medical facilities. They can offer structured therapy or simply provide comfort to patients. An absolute highlight of two of my psychiatric hospitalizations were the therapy animal visits. Pet Partners is the leading therapy animal non-profit program. Volunteers can have their dogs certified as therapy dogs by the Alliance of Therapy Dogs.

Psychiatric daytime and residential programs have also incorporated farm animals as part of daily living activities. Farm animals offer some of the same benefits of pet ownership. A few examples of the programs include Fountain Farms, Gould Farm, and Hopewell.

If you can't own a pet there are ways you can interact with animals up close. These include volunteering at a local shelter or even visiting animal sanctuaries such as the Wood Sanctuary, which I like to do.

Animals can be a wonderful part of life. They are an underutilized mental health intervention that could benefit many more. Research has shown their benefits, and anecdotal accounts are plentiful. They can ease the loneliness so many of us with mental illness suffer from, one of the most painful experiences of our illness. Animals can offer the support that we may lack and complement the support that we have. My personal experiences are similar to possibly millions of people. My Dude helped give me the gift of life when I struggled in the depths of my suicidal depression. He will forever be with me. "I carry his heart with me, I carry him in my heart. I am never without him."

Resources

Human Animal Bond Research Institute (HABRI): https://habri.org/
Human Animal Bond Literature Review: https://bit.ly/3azFqQX

Edited version published in *National Alliance on Mental Illness Blog*, Nov. 2020.

28
Coping with Mental Illness: What Not To Do
Katherine Ponte

I was recently discussing coping strategies for my bipolar disorder with my psychiatrist. I was pressing him for new ways to cope. He told me that most of his other patients also tend to look for *what to do*—a new medication or treatment method—but it is just as important to focus on *what not to do*.

I was interested in learning more about the experience of his other patients. After all, one of the most effective therapies has been learning I'm not alone, that other people have similar experiences. I wanted to know what he observed as the most common behaviors and habits that interfere with recovery and coping. Indeed, I learned that the obstacles I faced for years are actually fairly common: denial, ambivalence, ignorance and fear of stigma.

I could not help feeling regret as he listed them off. I realized that I had held myself back during all the years I denied the seriousness of my condition. In hindsight errors are obvious, but as I was experiencing the illness, I lacked the insight to make the right decisions. My doctor explained that these behaviors largely result from the "blind spots" that mental illness can create in our awareness. On top of that, stigma compounds the issue by limiting our perception of ourselves and the possibilities of living with mental illness.

Achieving recovery and coping with mental illness has required improvements to both my medical treatment and my interaction with my bipolar disorder. It has required increasing my awareness and coping by not doing behaviors created in response to stigma. Here are some of those harmful behaviors to avoid.

Denial

I stubbornly refused to accept my diagnosis of bipolar even though I knew something was wrong. That blind refusal took on many forms, including refusing all types of help. My treatment was needlessly delayed, which worsened my condition. I also refused to ask for help when it was clear that I needed it. The primary reason was fear of the consequences of being labeled as "mentally ill."

Dismissal

I often dismissed my family's input. I foolishly thought, "who are they to think they know better than me." But during many critical times they did know better. For example, my spouse has always been better than me at spotting signs of my hypomania. He can often see my blind spots. My refusals and dismissiveness also lessened my family's motivation to find me help. I didn't fully appreciate their efforts to help me, but looking back I know they had my best interest at heart.

Ignorance

I remained uninformed about my condition as a form of denial. I was worried that my suspicions, my health care provider's assessment and my family's concern would be confirmed if I became more informed about my condition. Ignorance made me a poor patient. I lacked the knowledge and impartial perspective to effectively assess and influence my treatment. I was sometimes combative when my doctor suggested a medication adjustment. I didn't know how to effectively express my treatment objectives and ask for medication alternatives. I wasn't self-aware enough to recognize the signs that my condition was deteriorating, and I needed to adjust to stay on track.

Non-adherence

I was non-adherent to my treatment plan a couple of times. I convinced myself that I was well and didn't need my medications. When my symptoms became less pronounced, I immediately thought I'd been cured. Without proper medical advice, I reduced and stopped taking my medication, which led to a serious manic episode and hospitalization. I now understand the consequences of stopping my medication without consulting my doctor.

Recklessness

I was impulsive and ignored my safety on a few occasions. In one instance, I was furious with the rapid weight gain, which is a side effect of the medication. I insisted that my doctor either reduce my dose or stop the medication completely. I got what I asked for, and I also got manic along with it. On another occasion, I hid my symptoms from my spouse

116

because I was worried I might be hospitalized. My condition worsened, and I ended up being hospitalized. I have learned to trust those closest to me and accept the help when it's offered.

Ambivalence

Even after accepting my diagnosis, I remained ambivalent about my treatment for many years. This led me to accept subpar treatment. I didn't ask if there were options, if things could be better. Due to my apathy, my spouse had to step in and make treatment decisions for me, which I ultimately resented. I would take my medication and attend therapy, but do little else. I'd take a fistful of anti-depressants and lie in bed all day waiting for some magical transformation. I didn't give the treatment the support that it needed to be effective.

For many, these behaviors are deeply ingrained. Addressing them may involve facing your own insecurities and hopelessness that stigma instills in us. But if we don't, we may limit our ability to fully adopt and benefit from new treatment strategies.

I learned the hard way that I was holding my recovery back. For over 15 years, I struggled. I had convinced myself that nothing would ever change, that nothing would ever work. I denied myself and my treatment the benefit of the doubt. Maybe things would have been different if the feeling of repeatedly losing hope wasn't so painful. The last time I reached out for help might have been my last, but I grasped hope once more and never let go. I won't ever let go again. It finally led me towards recovery and back to my family. I realized that not having hope was my greatest blind spot of all.

"Katherine's candid description of times when she more than once "got in her own way," possibly undermining her own treatment goals, is far from unusual and, I suspect, will sound familiar to many readers who struggle either first- or second-hand with chronic mental health conditions. By definition, it is awfully hard, if not almost impossible, to recognize blind spots. I applaud her candor and self-reflection." – Dr. Goldberg

Originally published in *National Alliance on Mental Illness Blog*, Jan. 25, 2020.

29

From Helicoptering to Collaborating:
Working on Recovery with Loved Ones
Katherine Ponte

Having a partner over-involved in your recovery plan can result in frustration, resentment, and confrontation. When you collaborate though, you can work as a team on your recovery.

I couldn't stand my spouse "helicoptering." It was part of his over-involvement in my care which disempowered, discouraged, infantilized and enraged me. I admit that at times my refusal to accept my condition, dismissiveness of his concerns, medical non-adherence and ambivalence left him no choice. Still, the helicoptering significantly contributed to my stress levels, which have always been a key trigger for my mania.

It felt like I was under constant surveillance. He'd hover over me, circle round, popup from behind, fly by. He saw impending mania in everything I said or did. I was disempowered as he and my former doctor took control of my treatment. He discouraged me by always expecting the worst, infantilized me by constantly watching over me, and enraged me when he didn't trust me. At the time, it strained our relationship as management of my condition became highly confrontational between the two of us. We both knew that the situation had grown untenable and that we had to address it to help me recover and to save our marriage from bipolar.

As I started to move towards stability and things got better, we recognized a few practices and changes that could help reach recovery quicker and better. These steps combined into a simple approach to help us work together constructively to address my condition and achieve recovery.

Establish guiding principles

We came up with a set of guiding principles that would define our shared involvement in my care. I recognized that my care was better with his involvement both one-on-one, and together with my clinician, as he has always been better at spotting signs of my hypomania than I have. We agreed that I would take control of my own care. I would set treatment goals, prioritize competing objectives and manage my condition. He and my clinician would play supporting roles, except when I was incapacitated. This approach allowed me to take more responsibility for outcomes. Perhaps most importantly, he and I both acknowledged each other's situation. He acknowledged how difficult it must be for me to live with my condition, and I acknowledged how difficult it must have been for him to do all that he could to help me when I didn't want to be helped.

Establish treatment objectives

It was important that I establish my own treatment objectives. I wanted to sleep less since I had been sleeping 14 hours a day. I wanted to lose weight because I was 70 pounds overweight. I wanted to pursue a career. My doctor and spouse recognized my objectives and did everything they possibly could to help me achieve them. My clinician adjusted my medication to cut my sleep time back to 9 hours a day, and put me on a stimulant to address daytime drowsiness. Reducing the dosage on one of my medications that hindered weight loss allowed me to shed the excess 70 pounds. My spouse did everything he could to help me plan and pursue a career.

Key treatment execution

I promised my spouse that I would be medically compliant and asked him to stop constantly checking in on me. My psychiatrist agreed to let me stay on my stimulant, which could create a risk of hypomania, if I reduced other hypomania risks in my life. I accepted the trade-off because the stimulant allowed me to be more functional in the daytime hours. I also agreed to take better care of myself. I started to work out at the gym with a trainer. My spouse kept me motivated by going to the gym with me. I now go to the gym four times a week. I also agreed to eat better, which my spouse strongly influenced. I now eat a healthy salad for dinner most nights. We also spend a lot of time in the country, which has been critical to my self-care. He encourages me and we do things together, which makes it easier to stay motivated and keep on track.

Triggers and relationship sensitivities

We openly identified and discussed my triggers to try to avoid them. These included my spouse's helicoptering and criticizing me for not doing more, and my not doing my fair of domestic duties. He explained to me that he couldn't stop watching over me, but that he would not do it so intrusively. I agreed to do more around the house even when I was depressed.

I also explained to him that I found some of the things he said to me to be triggering. When I disagreed with him, he might ask me if I was taking my meds or threaten to reach out to my doctor. He would ask "Are you amping up?" when he thought I was becoming hypomanic. He agreed to modify his behavior and words. Specifically, he agreed not to ask me if I was taking my medication when I disagreed with him, and to contact my doctor only under agreed circumstances (by email with a copy to me and only when I showed clear signs of hypomania). He also agreed to stop using the phrase "You're amping up." Now he says something like "I think you might not be well." It makes a big difference. These changes were important to me because they were connected to my past behavior and I wanted a fresh start, something that didn't remind me about the past.

Crisis preparation

We both agreed to do all that we could to avoid the next crisis after I had relapsed four times. The 911 calls and hospitalizations had been traumatizing to me, and my manic episodes had been traumatizing to him. So we both agreed to address signs of hypomania as quickly as possible. My key signs have always been preoccupation with social injustices, unusual stress, a fluster of creative activity, and in particular, reduced sleep. We address sleep disruption immediately. My doctor may make medication adjustments to get my sleep back on track and nip potential mania in the bud.

It's difficult for me to manage my bipolar, but it can also be very difficult for family members. The best approach to managing my bipolar has been a strong coalition between my psychiatrist, my spouse, and me, with me at the helm. I've never felt better. I've wrestled back control over my life from my bipolar.

Originally published in *bpHope*, May 29, 2019.

30
Learning to Take Care of Myself
Izzy Gonçalves

Over the two decades my spouse has struggled with bipolar disorder, I put aside my needs for hers. I have been her primary caregiver from the beginning. We have gone through five manic episodes and three hospitalizations, together. Each time required us to "rebuild" our home, back to stability and normalcy.

Since her first manic episode, I have put her needs for stability ahead of everything else in our life. I have been her monitor and guardian. I have helped her through her lows and pushed her to realize her potential. And I have often forgotten about myself in this process.

Over time, I learned this mentality was wrong and counterproductive. Because I gave up so much of myself, I resented my spouse. I grew distant from friends and family, in part due to the stigma of her illness and fear that they would not understand.

Between looking after my spouse and work, I had little, if any, time for other activities. I bottled up my emotions. I tried to numb myself. It seemed like the best defense mechanism when faced with a volatile situation, like one of my spouse's manic episodes. But stress and anxiety were always percolating and would intrude on me at work and in social interactions.

Eventually, my spouse found hope and the path to recovery. As she has taken more responsibility for her condition and life, it has made me realize the importance of caring for myself as well. She has encouraged me to do more for my health and enjoyment. So, I am taking care of my number one now — me.

Focusing on my self-care has been my own recovery process, one that has paralleled my spouse's. I think of it in terms of three components:

Redefining My Role as a Caregiver

I stopped feeling like my spouse's health was all on my shoulders. By letting go and allowing her to have more control of her treatment, I was able to transfer primary responsibility while still playing an important role in her care.

I stopped waiting for disaster to happen while recognizing the risks of future episodes. I learned more about how to manage and prepare for those risks. I learned more about her condition, triggers, symptom monitoring, coping strategies and prevention tools. It was essential to develop a strong "working relationship" with my spouse and her doctor.

I now feel less stress. I wait for signs of emotional swings instead of looking for them constantly. My spouse and I have an agreement that I can alert her and her doctor when I spot warning signs of a potential episode — and we have a plan if that happens.

For years, I couldn't help but partially blame myself for my spouse's early hospitalizations. I had made the 911 calls. Over time, I recognized that I hadn't had a choice, but the guilt lingered. And while she refused her diagnosis, she partially blamed me as well. But no more. Being a caregiver can be a very difficult situation, with lots of sacrifice and difficult choices. I have finally accepted that I did everything as best I could to help her. I also appreciate more and more that I am doing something special. And she agrees.

Prioritizing My Health

For years, my spouse's health took priority over all else. In particular, I put aside my own mental health to focus entirely on hers. After all, I was the stable one, the supporter. This was foolish. In fact, her episodes had been traumatic — for both of us.

I felt that our family, professional and social lives had been suspended. It caused me insecurity, anxiety and depression. And I did nothing about it. Finally, as my spouse became more focused on her treatment, she encouraged me to do the same for my emotional health. Now I have seen a therapist for years. It has given me great perspective on my life and armed me with coping strategies and tools to improve and protect my emotional health. It has also made me a better caregiver. Our discussions have enabled me to better understand her perspective, but also to prioritize my role in our relationship and my own life.

I have also focused on my physical health. As a caregiver, I often felt a lack of control over my circumstances. I was at the mercy of my spouse's illness, so I felt vulnerable. The emotional toll also affected my energy, strength and resilience. But I grew more positive and optimistic as I saw my therapist. It encouraged me to pursue well-being in other aspects of my life. I started to go the gym regularly. I focused on my diet. Over time, I reduced alcohol consumption. I started getting more sleep. These changes, very gradual at first, all give me a sense of control over my body and self.

Space

I have created space for myself not only in exercising but in a range of other activities like reading, spending more time outdoors and pursuing new hobbies. These activities allow me to engage with my own interests. They help define who I am beyond caregiving.

Creating this space is also establishing boundaries as a caregiver with your loved one. I admit this is an area where we continue to struggle, particularly with my spouse's mental illness advocacy, non-profit and entrepreneurial activities. It is easy to talk about mental illness all the time, which can be extremely draining. We need to take more mental illness time-outs. This can include agreeing to talk only about other subjects during dinner or parts of the weekend. Disengaging from the topic of mental illness can allow the mind to refresh and revisit the issues with more clarity and calm.

Additionally, creating space means engaging with other people. Part of coming to terms with my spouse's condition, and my caregiver role, has been to open up to friends, colleagues and family. I have re-engaged with relationships I had allowed stigma to quiet. I have removed the weight of stigma.

By talking about my experience, I have also discovered the shared experience of people dealing with similar issues in their lives. I personally have felt the power of support from other caregivers and loved ones.

Nurturing these relationships also helps create a network of support and understanding. This network can help keep out the forces of anxiety and depression. It also helps strengthen my role as a caregiver.

So take care of yourself. It is not at all selfish. In fact, it will make you an even better caregiver. But most importantly, it will help achieve the fulfillment and wellness you deserve.

Originally published in *National Alliance on Mental Illness Blog*, Jan. 23, 2020.

Part IV.
Specific Experiences

31
Learning from Past Manias
and Avoiding Future Relapses
Katherine Ponte

I was walking a tightrope, trying to stave off another episode. Then came my 4th relapse. Finally, it clicked: I needed to translate my personal history into a prevention plan. Here's how I did it.

I've been living with severe bipolar I disorder for over fifteen years. I've had five full-blown manic episodes. That's four relapses. After my first manic episode, I didn't think I'd have another. It was horrible—the episode, the shock, and the aftermath. I wanted to forget and leave it behind as soon as I could. It was too painful to recall those memories. I told myself it was a one-time event and to move on.

I liked being hypomanic, though. I *wanted* to be hypomanic—the optimal creative, energetic, and productive version of myself. I didn't appreciate that the downside of hypomania, for me, was how quickly it could escalate into mania. I failed to learn from my first experience. If I had evaluated what had happened, I might have been able to prevent the relapses or at least better manage them.

After I had my first relapse, I still didn't think it would happen again. After my second relapse, I had to accept that this was a reality of my illness. I knew that I had to avoid getting sick at all costs. I had to assess the damage and setback caused by each manic episode. It would take me no less than six months to recover from each hospitalization. To move forward with my life, the relapses had to end. I relied on medication, my doctor, and my spouse to keep from slipping.

I walked a tightrope for years, pushing to live a fuller life while avoiding a manic episode. Sometimes, motivated by a cause or project, I would find myself fully engaged and energized. I could feel the hypomania surge. A few times, when no one else stopped me, I cycled up to the edge, then slipped past the point of no return and into mania. I relapsed, and the process would start over.

It was only after my fourth relapse that the key missing piece sunk in. I finally realized that I had to be the most active participant in my care. I also had to reevaluate my entire treatment. If my treatment better

127

accommodated my creativity and drive, perhaps I wouldn't crave the high of hypomania. I couldn't rely only on my doctor and spouse to keep me in the safe zone. I needed to take ownership. But I also couldn't do it alone. I still needed the right medical treatment and family support, but I needed to be the team leader.

Taking ownership required me to face my prior episodes. I couldn't forget them. My relapses showed that I hadn't learned from my experiences. The answer to preventing relapse was in studying and learning from my history. Here I summarize the process I followed to translate my personal history into a prevention plan. I've organized it as a series of steps that might help others learn from their mental health episodes and sustain recovery.

Step 1 – Review the past

Document what happened from the beginning to the end of the manic episode.

- Create a timeline that documents the occurrence of triggers, mood changes, and the onset of symptoms such as behavior and sleep changes

- Gather feedback from witnesses, such as your significant other and doctors who observed the cycle and saw things you couldn't or don't remember

- Collect evidence from these episodes, including notable emails and writings

Step 2 – Analyze the patterns

If you have experienced multiple episodes, evaluate the recurring patterns between them. This history will help predict and curtail new episodes. These are some of the patterns I observed in my episodes.

- Prior to my triggers appearing, I was often in a state of deep depression.

- My triggers always involved issues of social injustice.

- Triggers manifested themselves in email missives, fixation on the news, religious preoccupation, and dismissal of other people's concerns.

- My main symptoms were racing thoughts and lack of sleep.

- Interests and habits became amplified to extreme levels. For example, lighting a candle from time to time morphed into lighting many candles all at once. An interest in saints intensified into a religious preoccupation.

- I escalated very quickly from triggering events to symptoms and then mania.

Step 3 – Develop rules based on the patterns

Identifying these patterns can help identify the onset of a new episode. Setting up rules of thumb based on historical experience can help defuse or manage an episode. Below are a couple of the rules I developed.

- If I experience any of my usual signs of hypomania, I should let my doctor and spouse know immediately.

- Having a sleepless night is a key sign of cycling up for me. I should contact my doctor, who might adjust medication to help me sleep.

- Certain behaviors that became amplified when manic were OK in moderation, but should be monitored. For example, lighting a candle shouldn't be cause for alarm, but if it persisted and became obsessive, it was likely a reliable sign that I was cycling up.

- Try to remove triggers. I learned to turn off the news when news events started to wear on me.

- If I feel consumed by a social mission or issue, I try to step away. Recognize that many are issues are out of my control. Discuss my preoccupation with my doctor and spouse.

- If I have been stewing over something all day, I try to get out of the house and/or talk to a friend, go for a walk, or hit the gym.

Step 4 – Assign responsibilities

For me, recovery has been a team effort with doctors and family. Along with developing rules, we also assigned responsibilities for actions based on these rules.

- As a witness to my previous episodes, my spouse has a great sense for early indicators that I am cycling up. He has my blessing to contact my doctor when he sees me showing these signs. I asked him to communicate with my doctor by text or email with a copy to me so that I am not excluded and there's no miscommunication.

- We must trust each other. I know that my doctor will be objective and not accept my spouse's word as the authority. He does his best to evaluate everyone. We all need to be open to each other's perspectives and trust that our common goal is my recovery.

Step 5 – Implement the plan

In the past, I had often resisted and resented my doctor and spouse taking control when I started to cycle up. Now, I maintain control and allow myself to be a partner in my treatment by putting in place a plan that provides for different scenarios.

- I authorized my spouse to speak with my doctor, using the protocol for communication mentioned above.

- I recognize that my spouse needs to take control when I'm no longer in a position to make lucid decisions for myself. I have prepared formal instructions for this scenario, but I should better formalize them in an Advance Psychiatric Directive.

My doctor, Dr. Joseph Goldberg, who has expertise in bipolar disorder, recently offered a good driving analogy to understand the value of partners in care. Someone with mental illness should recognize that they can't always observe the risks of a brewing manic episode on their own. Sometimes, we know that there are "blind spots", like in driving, in our perception of these risks, so we are careful to navigate away from them. At other times, we mistakenly ignore a blind spot and get into an accident. Our ability to realize blind spots exist when we don't see them, and to ask for assistance in identifying them, helps to keep us healthy and safe. We need partners in care to point out the blind spots we don't see.

Originally published in *bpHope*, Jan. 2, 2020.

32
Turning Suicidal Ideation into Hope
Katherine Ponte

From an early age, I was driven by conventional markers of success: academic and professional accomplishment and most importantly, financial wealth. As the child of immigrant parents, these markers were particularly important to me. I saw money as a measure that transcended cultural barriers and norms. Enough of it would establish my worth in our adopted home.

So, I worked diligently toward this dream. I excelled in school. I graduated high school early and completed college and then law school. First, I was a lawyer, and then, I wanted to become an investment banker, so I could have even greater earning power.

My early career was a life of work and nothing else. I would proudly work 14-16 hours a day, including weekends. I'd brag about how I could pull all-nighters. I wanted to be a workaholic. I saw others in the same field working just as hard as I was. I came to believe that this was what being successful was all about. Slowly, as I tired of being exhausted all the time, watching the years of my youth pass by, I started to change my views.

My MBA program and early exposure to investment banking only cemented my growing dissatisfaction. How I felt forced me to confront the realities of this career goal. All my life I had worked toward a dream that made me miserable. My ambitions were deflated. And I didn't have a backup plan, so I wasn't able to redirect my energy elsewhere. Depression took over. It took away all my hope. Then I had my first manic episode. That manic episode combined with several more in the coming years swallowed me up and hijacked my life.

From Dreams to Suicidal Ideation

Suddenly, I was "bipolar." To me, this could have no place in my success. I tried to dismiss the first manic episode and the diagnosis. I convinced myself that it was a one-time anomaly and not a part of me. I refused to come to terms with my bipolar disorder. This refusal would lead me toward self-destruction.

I started to believe the limitations society projected onto me. I accepted society's stigmas toward mental illness and turned them into self-stigma. I no longer believed I could achieve success or have a high-powered career. I felt like a complete failure, like I had disappointed my family, especially my spouse and parents. I was embarrassed and ashamed.

I took preemptive strikes to protect myself from other people's reactions toward the "ill" me.

I pushed people away. I refused help. I stopped communicating with my spouse. I communicated with my parents only enough for them to know I was alive. I refused to take calls from friends. I told them to leave me alone. It was a way of staying in control. I completely retreated and isolated myself.

I was hopeless and helpless for many years. I felt I had no reason to live. I wanted to escape my pain and suffering. I was convinced I could never make it stop. I was left considering suicide as a way to fix the situation. In my head, it was the only way. My suicidal ideation gradually increased over the years. It took over my thoughts and my mind. I reached a point where I spent more time thinking of reasons to die than to live.

Finally Finding Hope and Meaning

My last hospitalization due to a manic episode gave me a jolt of realization. I happened to learn about peer-based support, and I was exposed to examples of other people living well with mental illness. These people defined success not with money, but with what made them happy. I found a network of peers, a community, that was diverse and vibrant, and successful in many ways. They inspired me. They helped set me on a new path to find meaning in my life and combat my suicidal ideations. These are the three principles I learned along the way.

- Career success is doing something that makes you happy.It has been long established that helping others benefits both the recipient and the giver. This is my life philosophy now.Every day I wake up in the morning hoping to inspire just one person that recovery from mental illness is real.

    I developed ForLikeMinds with this goal. It may not make me successful the way I used to define it, but it brings me immeasurable wealth. I also love volunteering with my local

NAMI-NYC affiliate and writing for the NAMI Blog. Knowing that I am in some way contributing to people's understanding of mental illness and helping others adds true meaning in my life.

- There is no happiness or success without strong relationships. For years, I distanced and isolated myself from my family and friends. I was too consumed with my own pain and suffering to realize what I was doing to others. I didn't speak to some of my friends for five or more years. I never fathomed that they needed me as much as I needed them.

  When I reached recovery, I apologized to my family and friends. I realized that my family never stopped loving me. I was wrong to think otherwise. My friends focused on the fact that I was back and not why I had retreated. Of course, many of my former friends did not take me back, but the most important ones did.

  I wouldn't have experienced such long periods of suicidal ideation if I hadn't isolated myself. As I emerged from suicidal ideation and recovered, I realized the true meaning of the love of family and caring friendships. Now I nurture and cherish them, and they help keep me well. They come above all else.

- To live well with mental illness, you have to understand your mental illness.

  It has taken me a long time to come to terms with the fact that I have mental illness—that it's a chronic disease that will not go away. But it also doesn't mean I can't have a fulfilling life. It required a lot of adjustment, but it was critical to learn how to live well with mental illness rather than letting the struggle of it take over my life.

I also had to better understand the risks—especially suicide—of bipolar disorder and not be complacent or dismissive of them. I have grown to respect the seriousness of my illness and take more responsibility for it, such as prioritizing treatment.

I've learned to transform suicidal thinking into thoughts of hope. I can now manage and cope with these thoughts and be empowered by them to help others. Mental illness may take a lot away from us, but the struggle can bring us closer to understanding the meaning of our lives. Now, I have many reasons to live for. I have hope to share, and I want to share it with as many people as possible.

Originally published in *National Alliance on Mental Illness Blog*, Sep. 11, 2019.

33
Suicide: Saving Lives Now and Beyond
Katherine Ponte

Suicide is a public health crisis. Suicide rates rose 25% in the U.S. from 1999 to 2016. In 2018, nearly 50,000 people died by suicide, around 11 million seriously thought about it, about 3 million made a plan and over 1 million attempted suicide. These numbers represent immeasurable tragic losses to human life, friends, family and society.

There is an urgent need to address the causes. Most suicide prevention programs focus on the now — the risk factors, which are essential. However, these programs should also focus on protective factors to have a longer lasting impact on those vulnerable to suicide.

What are the Risk Factors of Suicide?

Here are some of the primary risk factors for suicide, which may help us identify at-risk populations and individuals.

1. Previous attempt: The leading suicide risk factor is a prior suicide attempt.

2. Triggers: These can include a wide range of significant events, especially relationship problems and unemployment. Additionally, a history of child abuse, including bullying or sexual abuse, traumatic brain injury, chronic pain and chronic health conditions may heighten suicide risk.

3. Mental illness: It is estimated that nearly 90% of people worldwide who die by suicide have a mental illness. However, only about 50% of people who die by suicide in the U.S. are actually diagnosed with mental illness.

4. Substance abuse: People who are dependent on alcohol or use drugs have a 10-14 times greater suicide risk than the general population. This risk is even more significant when a there is a co-occurrence of substance use disorders and mental illness.

5. Impulsivity: One study found that more than 50% of suicide attempts were impulsive. Other studies have found that up to 50% of those who attempt suicide decide to do so within minutes to an

hour before acting.

6. Access to firearms: a key suicide prevention measure is to reduce access to firearms, which can significantly increase suicide risk.

7. Ethnicity/race: the highest rates across ages are among American Indian/Alaska Native and white populations.

8. Sexual orientation/gender identity: LGB youth are almost five times as likely to attempt suicide compared to heterosexual youth. Transgender adults are at even higher risk with 40% reporting a suicide attempt in their lifetime.

A combination of therapy and medication can help address some of these risk factors. But we also need to think about how we can protect the most vulnerable in other ways.

What are Protective Factors for Suicide?

We often take a "reactive" approach to suicide risk. We identify risk factors and watch for warning signs. But sometimes, by the time warning signs are visible to others, it's too late. An additional approach that may increase our impact is to identify protective factors that can help shield individuals from becoming at-risk in the first place.

Each person has their own "reasons for living" and recognizing them can be life-saving. The Reasons for Living Scale identifies possible protective factors for suicide, including meaningful relationships with friends and family, survival instincts, excitement about future plans, and the belief that happiness is an important part of life. These protective factors can not only reduce suicide risk, they can be good for general well-being and foster happiness.

During my extended periods of suicidal ideation in my struggles with bipolar, I would often reflect on my reasons for living. I felt that a suicide attempt or death would hurt my family too much, and I would not want them to suffer. I imagined the reaction of my spouse who had stuck by me. I imagined how my parents would take it after lovingly raising me and always being there for me. I imagined them heartbroken and filled with inconsolable grief and blaming themselves. I even thought of my cat, Dude, who never left my side in my darkest moments.

I also feared death. I'd hear examples of suicide in the news and it would heighten my own thoughts, but I ultimately couldn't go through with it. I was scared of dying and knew deep down that I wanted to live.

As I moved towards recovery, I discovered that I did have reasons for living and recovery itself gave me even more reasons. My overwhelming pain and suffering, hopelessness and self-stigma had blinded me to these reasons and possibilities. I finally reached a point where I no longer thought of suicide, but instead recognized all the good in my life.

I realized that I had caring and loving social support, which I learned to accept. While this may not be for everyone, I also — very skeptically at first — learned to have greater faith in a higher power to "take care" of the things I could not control and help me in times of need. I personally believe this higher power can take different forms with people - religious, spiritual, philosophical, scientific, social, etc. As my condition improved, my hope grew. Hope bolstered my belief that I had a future worth living, which I had to seize day-by-day. It would be a future supported by my friends and family.

We need to start coming together and **speaking** to each other more. We need to nurture and develop protective factors, especially among those closest to us. We need to stop missing opportunities to save lives through more caring and loving action among and between each other.

We can stop suicide, but we have to do it together. Suicide is not only an individual tragedy, it is a collective tragedy, our tragedy.

Resources

National Suicide Prevention Lifeline: https://suicidepreventionlifeline.org/ - 1-800-273-8255
American Foundation for Suicide Prevention: https://afsp.org/
Crisis Text Line: https://www.crisistextline.org/ - text HOME to 741741 (24/7)
The Trevor Project: https://www.thetrevorproject.org/ - 866-488-7386 (24/7), Text START to 678678
The Veterans Crisis Line: https://www.veteranscrisisline.net/get-help/chat - 800-273-8255 and press 1 (24/7), Text 838255 (24/7)
Vets4Warriors: https://www.vets4warriors.com/
SAMHSA'S National Helpline (Substance Abuse): https://www.samhsa.gov/find-help/national-helpline - 800-662-HELP (4357) (24/7)

The National Alliance on Mental Illness: https://bit.ly/3fblmFS
The Jed Foundation: https://www.jedfoundation.org/
Speaking of Suicide: https://www.speakingofsuicide.com/
Medscape: https://bit.ly/339ULVh
CDC Suicide Resources:
https://www.cdc.gov/violenceprevention/suicide/resources.html

Suicide education

LivingWorks Applied Suicide Intervention Skills Training (ASIST):
https://www.livingworks.net/
LivingWorks safe TALK: https://www.livingworks.net/safetalk
QPR Gatekeeper Training for Suicide Prevention: https://bit.ly/3hZpZo1

Originally published in the *National Alliance on Mental Illness Blog*, Sep. 10, 2020.

34
My Reality During a Psychotic Episode
Katherine Ponte

The end of the world was near. I was a prophet. I had to save us from ourselves.

It was 2006. I had been living with untreated severe bipolar I disorder for over six years. I became psychotic trying to understand our often-nonsensical world: death and destruction from religious conflict, murderous terrorist plots and attacks and countless social injustices. My inability to rationalize such irrational behavior took me to a place I'd never been before. Reality turned into delusion.

I Thought the World Was Ending

At the time, it seemed like every five minutes there was a breaking news alert. I have never been able to stand by and not act on an issue I felt strongly about. I raised the alarm with friends and family, emailing as many as I could about what was happening in the world, about my concerns and fears. Almost no one replied.

A couple wrote back to ask if I was okay, but no one talked about my concerns. I contacted many media outlets to share my carefully researched and documented concerns. Nobody cared. No one would listen to me. So I turned, as my mother always had, to God. I prayed. I prayed to the many saints of my Catholic faith to intercede on my behalf.

I anxiously turned to CNN hoping for a change in news. Nothing. All was the same. I then turned to other faiths: Islam, Judaism, Buddhism, Hinduism. I bought various religious books and articles. I built a large altar on my living room table. My husband dismissed it. He had known me to be eccentric before. I visited countless houses of worship to pray, adopting other expressions of faith. I would talk to parishioners, leave "please save the world" notes in donation boxes. I once again anxiously turned to CNN hoping to hear the world had been saved in the latest breaking news. Nothing. All was still the same.

I Believed I Could Save the World

After the other religions didn't work, I turned to the most mysterious, even feared, religion I knew—Candomble—a practice I learned about during my time in Brazil. I turned to Iansa, the orixa (spirit goddess) of thunder and storms. I dressed in red from head to toe. I placed a tall statue of her atop my altar.

I called on her to help me. I praised her, worshipped her and prayed to her. I even made offerings of chocolates, wine and money to her. I would blare trance-like music, and dance around my apartment with an indigenous rain stick trying to invoke Iansa. And still no change. The CNN breaking news alerts of tragedy and disaster continued.

I had a very difficult time falling asleep as images filled my head. All I could see in my mind were black mushroom clouds with darkened air swirling around. Music blared continually through my apartment from about 9am-9pm, until my husband came home. I knew he wouldn't understand any of it, and I didn't want him to stop me.

I Found Signs Everywhere

I empathized with John Lennon's "Imagine." I played it on continuous repeat. I visited the Imagine Mosaic in Central Park throughout the day and left peace offerings. One time, I left 100 or so copies of Kahlil Gibran's "On Friendship." I wanted people in the world to be friends with each other. I left candles, prayer beads, saints, objects of every religion.

I agonized that I was the only one who could see the world was ending. I played CNN nonstop. I never turned it off, not even when I slept, because I didn't want to miss the good news when it finally came.

I had begun sleeping on the couch just to be near the TV. But it was always the same. I was beginning to feel like a failure, but I knew that I could not stop. I was being guided by a greater power. I saw signs everywhere. In music, poems, books, billboards, even in garbage. I brought debris home to add to my altar.

Then, the final sign happened... a terrorist plot in Toronto foiled. My roots. A place that I'd always bragged represented cultural and religious unity. If it could happen there of all places, it could happen again anywhere. A bright light streamed through my window, and words filled my mind. It was God. I quickly wrote His message. My mission was to continue. I was not to be deterred. I shared this message with everybody

I knew, emailing it as widely as possible. I left copies at the Imagine Mosaic.

I Considered Myself a Prophet

It all culminated on one windy, thunderous night. I was Iansa fully possessed. I danced wildly in a trance-like state blaring music. I wore red markings on my face with a rain stick in one hand and swinging an old hammer in the other. I hurled my religious altar through the room, except Iansa. I swung that hammer like a bat at CNN. It no longer mattered what it said, I knew the ending. I ripped the blinds in my apartment down. I stuck notes to my windows—my message to outsiders.

My apartment was a disaster, completely trashed. I had blocked my front door, so my husband barged in through the back door. He was shocked. He held me tight, asking me what was wrong. I pushed him away. No one could stop me. But I was also afraid. John Lennon had been a prophet, and he was killed, and I might be killed too. They wanted to silence me.

My husband called 911. I was restrained and hauled off to the hospital.

I Finally Saw Reality

During my four-week hospital stay, all I could think of was getting back to my mission. Evil forces hospitalized me to stop me because I was getting closer to achieving my mission. A month later, I returned home. I immediately flushed all my medication down the toilet. I ran to the Imagine Mosaic. I yelled as loud as I could that people had to listen to me. I begged them to listen. Someone called 911. An ambulance arrived shortly. I was taken back to the hospital where I stayed another month. I was very closely monitored.

As the medications began to take effect. I very sadly started to realize that I was not Iansa, that I was not a prophet. I was just a very sick person.

I remain convinced to this day that I became psychotic trying to make sense of our world. I spoke to my doctor recently about it. He told me that real events are often what trigger psychotic episodes. People with mental illness are said to be highly empathetic and compassionate. Maybe that's what heightened my sensitivity to what was going on in the world. I've seen other examples, though not as extreme as mine. One time, someone in my support group whispered in my ear, "I can't watch the news, it makes me sick." I said, "me too." But for us, it really does. My psychotic experience may be unique, but the fact that it's grounded in reality doesn't seem to be all that unique.

Now when I come across a person who seems as if they might be delusional, I don't walk away. I lean in and listen carefully. I understand where they're coming from.

Originally published in *National Alliance on Mental Illness Blog*, Jun. 12, 2019.

35
Preventing and Preparing for a
Mental Health Crisis
Katherine Ponte

My experience during my crisis made me feel worse than my illness itself. Three armed police officers and two paramedics pounded on my door, entered my small apartment, checked my vitals, strapped me into a wheelchair, forcibly removed me from my home, and escorted me to a siren-blaring ambulance. I was shocked and confused. I yelled. I cried. I was terrified. I felt like I was being imprisoned.

I was involuntarily admitted to a chaotic psychiatric emergency room where I was isolated from my family and interviewed alone. I was then placed on a gurney and forcibly medicated multiple times. For two days, I was confined to a gurney in a psychiatric emergency room corridor before being admitted to the inpatient unit. I was deemed to be a danger to myself or others. It was embarrassing and disempowering. It was the ultimate loss of control.

Sadly, this is what a psychiatric crisis can look like for many people living with mental illness.

In 2016, 5.5 million people with mental, behavioral and neurodevelopmental disorders visited the emergency room. Mental illnesses are the third most common cause of hospitalization in the U.S. And for many living with severe mental illness, the first significant treatment experience is hospitalization, which is what happened to me.

My spouse and I were completely unprepared for a mental health crisis. The experience had long-lasting and traumatizing effects, magnified by how unprepared and uninformed we were. It's essential to recognize the possibility of a crisis and be prepared, while also working to prevent it. Unfortunately, the health care process is not always logical, orderly or friendly. And we certainly lacked the awareness and health education to be better prepared for it.

With that in mind, here is my advice based on my experience to help with crisis prevention and planning.

Planning in Advance

Early signs of an impending crisis

Knowing the early signs of an episode is key to planning for a crisis. For people living with bipolar disorder, reduced sleep is a telltale sign of hypomania (an elevated mood that is similar to mania, but less severe). My spouse usually notices it before I do and calls my psychiatrist immediately. A quick medication adjustment has on multiple occasions contained my hypomania before it escalates to mania. My spouse's involvement is important as I often lack insight or am unaware when I start to become symptomatic. Other preventative measures are always taking my medication and at the appropriate doses, and abstaining from substance use. My past episodes provide me with invaluable insight into possible future episodes.

Psychiatric Advance Directive (PAD)

You should talk about a potential crisis with your caregiver in advance. The completion of a PAD provides the perfect opportunity to do so. A PAD is a legal tool that allows you to state your treatment preferences in advance of a crisis. In the event we become incapacitated, it will speak for us indicating our preferred representative, preferred hospital, least favorite treatment, preferred medications, etc. It can be very empowering to have a PAD as you retain some control over your treatment even in times of crisis. It also allows caregivers to ask about your preferences, which may lead to enhanced family relationships. And it helps caregivers who at the time of a crisis may otherwise struggle trying to determine what their loved one might want. Standard forms can help you prepare your own PAD.

Privacy Issues

In some cases, health care providers are prohibited from sharing our treatment information with our caregivers unless we grant permission. This can be particularly frustrating to a caregiver during a crisis. It is essential for caregivers to talk about privacy issues beforehand, including what information you are comfortable with them having access to. It might be helpful to specify these permissions in a written waiver.

Alternatives to Hospitalization

Peer Respite

A less familiar crisis option is a peer respite. A peer respite is defined as "a voluntary, short-term, overnight program that provides community-based, non-clinical crisis support" in an environment that feels more like a home than a treatment setting. These facilities are staffed and operated by peers. Research shows that "guests" were 70% less likely to use inpatient or emergency services. A peer respite might be a helpful option to address an emerging crisis before it reaches emergency stage.

Outpatient Program

In a hospital setting, many hospitals have an adult outpatient or partial hospital program. In these programs, a person lives at home while engaging with services. Participation may be voluntary or mandated by court order. It may also precede or follow an inpatient hospitalization. The program is meant to ensure that a patient is stable and also facilitates their transition back into the community under hospital staff supervision. It also seeks to reduce or avoid future hospitalizations. The typical program lasts two weeks.

Emergency Engagement

Crisis Intervention Teams (CIT)

As an alternative to calling 911 in a mental health crisis, a person may call a CIT. According to CIT International, a CIT is a "community partnership of law enforcement, mental health and addiction professionals, individuals who live with mental illness and/or addiction disorders, their caregivers, and advocates." These support teams are present in over 2,700 communities across the U.S. CITs are widely considered a best practice model in law enforcement. There are several benefits to CITs, including the reduction of arrests and need for additional mental health services.

Another alternative is a mobile crisis team (MCT). A mobile crisis team of mental health care providers can attend to a person in need and conduct medical assessments. It may be helpful to research CITs or MCTs in your area and have their contact numbers handy to prepare for a potential crisis.

911

Calling 911 is the most elevated, and potentially contentious, course of action. I was angry with my spouse for years for calling 911. I blamed him for my hospitalization. I was embarrassed and ashamed that my neighbors may have witnessed the events. In fear of a repeat experience, I was afraid to ask for help, which ultimately led to two subsequent hospitalizations. As I became well, I came to appreciate my spouse's predicament at the time. I think we would have handled the crisis much differently and avoided the need for a 911 call if we had been prepared. It might be helpful to include in your crisis plan guidance on the circumstances in which to call 911.

Hospitalization

If the circumstances allow, it might be helpful to seek a second opinion from a psychiatrist when facing the difficult choice of whether to receive inpatient care. When hospitalization is deemed the best course of action, a patient is typically admitted to a psychiatric emergency room. It may be helpful to know in advance that it can be chaotic and a shortage of beds is common. And that, upon admission, a patient is continuously monitored. It is worth discussing with the doctor if they have admitting privileges or other relationship at a hospital that may be suitable. If so, they may be able to facilitate the admission process.

Crisis was the most difficult mental health experience for my spouse and me. If we knew how to prevent a crisis, how to handle one and what to expect, our experiences and outcomes could have been better. I now know that there are alternatives to calling 911. I pray that I never experience another crisis, but if I do, I am certain it will not be as traumatizing. Getting help should make you feel better, not worse.

References

Psychiatric Advance Directive (PAD): https://www.nrc-pad.org

Originally published in *National Alliance on Mental Illness Blog*, Dec. 9, 2019.

36
That Time in the Psych Ward
Katherine Ponte

I have been hospitalized three times. I was given heavily sedating medication much of the time, but I will never forget what I went through. Each time, I was in crisis, at my life's lowest point, looking for a path forward. I felt powerless and despondent. But I was treated like I was a threat to others' safety, as if I had done something terribly wrong. Instead of receiving care, my experiences left me scarred, stalled and aimless for years afterwards.

I Needed Treatment, Not Sedation

My last psychiatric hospitalization was the most painful. I arrived, strapped into a wheelchair, to a chaotic psychiatric emergency room. They separated me from my husband to interview me. After my intake, they placed me on a gurney and forcibly medicated me.

I was left on that gurney in the corridor of a psychiatric ER for two days before an inpatient-psychiatric bed became available. I couldn't sleep or rest. Another psych patient wailed constantly. I was in internal crisis, yet there was crisis all around me. The last thing I can remember from my experience in the ER was being forcibly medicated one more time.

Once admitted to the inpatient ward, I awoke to find myself in leather restraints. There was no one there to explain where I was or why I was being detained or subdued. I didn't know what was happening. I was alone.

As I slowly gained awareness of myself and my surroundings, it became clear that we were under constant watch. The staff was concerned that we were potentially dangerous to ourselves and others. Everything in the psych ward was violence- and suicide-proof. Even the personal belongings our loved ones brought were carefully checked. I had never been violent or suicidal before in my life. I started thinking: "Am I really *this* ill?" "Am I really violent and suicidal?" The severity of my illness and all that it meant, the stigma, started to sink in.

I Needed Help, Not Imprisonment

Treatment seemed to focus on immediate stabilization, rather than long-term health. I saw my assigned doctor infrequently, and more often I saw a resident. I couldn't see my outside doctor. I was placed on a new medication regimen. I was highly sedated for most of my stay. Many patients never left their room, and others spent the day walking loops around the ward. I never once saw a nurse in my room.

They kept us on a lock-down. I was never allowed to go outside, not even with an escort. Security guards roamed the floors. I also faced other restrictions, including suspension of computer and phone privileges, in-room confinement and solitary confinement to a seclusion room.

At one point, my condition significantly deteriorated, and I fell into a severe manic state. Two security guards picked me up and dragged me to a seclusion room furnished with only a thin red mattress on the floor. They wrapped my arm tightly around my back, pinned me to the floor, and then forcibly medicated me. They left me in a locked room for hours as a guard watched me through a small wire-glass window. When they released me, they placed me on around-the-clock surveillance for a week. They watched me even as I slept.

I Needed Support, Not Isolation

I desperately needed love, comfort and support from my family during my stay, but it was difficult to stay connected with them by phone or in person. There were no phones in the rooms. There were only a couple of payphones located in the hallway. As a policy, staff did not answer calls, only patients could answer. Often when a patient answered a call from my mother, they would tell her that they didn't know me, I was not there or they couldn't find me. There was no way to leave a message. Each time this happened, my mother worried that something might be wrong. She was often unable to reach me for days.

No visits were allowed in patient rooms, out of a fear that we might injure our loved ones. All visits had to occur in full view of clinicians, security and other patients and their visitors. It was more than a bit uncomfortable for my spouse and me to express our heartfelt emotions at this sensitive time in public view. Even a hug felt awkward when the person next to you had no visitors, which is often the case in the psych ward. These should be among the most private moments families have together, when a loved one is at their worst lows.

Visiting hours were three hours shorter per day for the psych ward than "regular" patients. Did we need less love, compassion and human contact? Were we somehow less worthy or important than "regular" patients?

This Needs to Change

I returned home after each one of my hospitalizations severely depressed. I was too demoralized to appreciate that I was discriminated against. At times, I was made to feel like a criminal being punished, a danger to society. I felt it was all my fault for getting sick in the first place. I felt that I deserved the treatment that I received. I was at a top hospital. This perception fed off the social stigma I already experienced and certainly did not help my recovery.

These inpatient experiences traumatize me to this day. We need to focus on how it can be better, to turn psychiatric hospitalization into a constructive turning point towards recovery. The only positive memory I have was of an occupational therapist from my last hospitalization. She treated patients with genuine care and affection. She designed programs not only to occupy us, but to inspire us to get better. She emphasized the power of peer support. She showed me my first example of a high functioning person with mental illness. She planted a seed that my fellow patients and I, struggling as we were, could get better.

I like to imagine a psych ward staffed with empathetic professionals like that therapist, and how much better the experience could be. She helped me get to where I am today, because she cared and shared tools to help me.

It felt like this is what a recovery-oriented psych ward should be like all the time:

> *A place that helps sick people recover, as a hospital should.*

> *A place that doesn't treat you like a violent criminal because you have mental illness.*

> *A place that shows compassion for how hard it is to go through a mental health crisis.*

A place that gives you treatment, care and support rather than sedation, isolation and discrimination.

Originally published in *National Alliance on Mental Illness Blog*, Mar. 11, 2019.

Part V.
Specific Communities

37
Suicide Prevention for College Students
John MacPhee and Katherine Ponte

Every year, over two million high school graduates start college. This is a proud moment for so many. These students are entering adulthood and taking the next step in their life. The risk of suicide may be the furthest thing from their minds, yet it is a growing reality on college campuses. In fact, it is now the second leading cause of death among people aged 10-43 in the U.S. Indeed, graduating is a proud moment and college is an exciting time but as these figures show it's also an anxious and vulnerable time. This risk requires a lot more attention.

Some of the attributes that may indicate risk include having a mental illness or substance use disorder. A 2018 study found that at any time within the last 12 months, 41% of students felt so depressed that it was difficult to function and 62% felt overwhelming anxiety. It is also estimated that one in five college students has a substance use disorder. Additional risk factors include relationship problems, a crisis in the prior two weeks, physical health problems, legal troubles, loss of housing and financial challenges.

Fortunately, there are actions that families, students and colleges can take to lower the risk of suicide.

What Families Can Do

The signs of depression in youth may resemble typical teenage angst. If family members have a feeling that something might be wrong, they should address any concerns as soon as possible. This will increase the likelihood of early recognition and diagnosis of an issue and improve treatment outcomes.

Families should also encourage teens and young adults to talk about any mental health challenges they are experiencing, including and especially suicidal behavior, with a counselor, family member or trusted adults. Families can let loved ones know that they would be supportive and receptive to discussing these more intimate and troubling concerns, and can help them get treatment. Fear of overreaction or misunderstanding is a key reason why some students may be reluctant to speak to families.

For young adults starting college who have a pre-existing mental health condition, they should create a college transition plan, including treatment continuity when on campus. Having a plan can better prepare students for the additional mental health stressors they may encounter in college.

It might also help for parents and families to maintain contact with the campus counseling center. Family members can provide helpful information on any relevant history that might evidence a suicide risk. However, privacy rules prevent counselors from sharing a student's treatment history with family. Obtaining HIPAA and FERPA waivers from your loved one, preferably at the start of the school year, may allow parents and family members to access important information to help support their loved one.

More generally, families can model and talk to their young adult about the importance of self-care, and where to go on campus for emotional or academic support. Parents can connect with other parents via parent portals, parent councils, Facebook groups and online forums such as ForLikeMinds to discuss ways to get involved. And they can advocate for resources and programming on their student's campus that address mental health.

What Students Can Do

Students are in a unique position to take control, advocate and watch out for their mental health and the mental health of their peers. Learning how to recognize the warning signs of mental health issues and how to help, including how to talk to peers, practice self-care, manage emotions, access help and learn how to be a better support for others are all ways students can have a positive impact.

Talking is critical. This is especially important if a student notices or has a gut feeling that another student is struggling. It is also more likely that a student will report emotional distress and suicidal ideation to another student rather than to an older adult. The JED Foundation has helpful videos to guide students through the conversation, called the Seize the Awkward campaign. On-campus student mental health groups may also be a good resource, such as NAMI on Campus. Students can also advocate for resources and programming on their campus.

Practicing self-care is critically important to stress management. This includes: engaging in social activities with good friends, having appropriate "me time," getting enough sleep and physical activity and seeking help when needed.

What Colleges Can Do

Colleges and universities have a unique opportunity to promote student mental health. JED's "Comprehensive Approach to Mental Health Promotion and Suicide Prevention for Colleges and Universities" describes what a college can do to help foster a mental health safety net for students.

Identify students at risk: It is important to identify students with mental health concerns, alcohol and other drug abuse problems, and any other students who are at risk for suicide before they are in crisis. This includes supporting the transition to college for incoming students with mental health histories, providing robust screening opportunities at multiple touch points in the student experience and training campus community members to identify, reach out to and refer students at risk.

Promote social connectedness: Research has shown that supportive social relationships and feeling connected to campus, family and friends are protective factors that can help lower suicide risk. This area includes core objectives aimed at promoting inclusiveness on campus: identifying and reaching out to disconnected and isolated students and supporting connectedness among traditionally marginalized or higher-risk student groups.

Increase help-seeking behavior: Ideally, students will be comfortable with and knowledgeable about asking for help. However, it's important to promote help-seeking by reducing the burden of stigma associated with mental health problems and increasing access to mental health resources and support.

Provide substance abuse and mental health services: Providing adequate, on-site access to mental health prevention support and direct services is the backbone of a college mental health system. On-campus services should include basic primary care and mental health and crisis support.

Follow crisis management procedures: Crisis management includes access to immediate emergency services on campus or in the community

155

and local or national crisis resources, as well as policies that protect and support students during a time of crisis. Additionally, there should be an appropriate institutional response to student suicide, death or other emergency.

Develop life skills: Supporting life skills education is a valuable strategy for helping students cope with life's stressors, make wise lifestyle choices, foster resilience and achieve academic success. This area includes promotion of emotional and interpersonal awareness and education about the links between emotional and physical wellness, and how they impact academic success.

Many families have experienced the tragedy of a loved one's loss at a time when they were filled with promise. We may never know what led these students to die by suicide, but that cannot hold us back from trying to prevent these tragedies. We need to acknowledge and address this growing problem. In fact, we must all work together — families, students, colleges and our society — to find answers and solutions.

John MacPhee, BA, MBA, MPH is the executive director and CEO of JED (jedfoundation.org). He is passionate about supporting young adults in their transition to adulthood. John advises several organizations including the S. Jay Levy Fellowship for Future Leaders at City College, Trek Medics, Crisis Text Line, the Health Policy and Management Department at the Mailman School of Public Health, and HIV Hero. John received The Allan Rosenfield Alumni Award for Excellence in the field of public health from the Joseph L. Mailman School of Public Health at Columbia University.

Originally published in *National Alliance on Mental Illness Blog*, Sep. 23, 2020.

38

Parents and their College Child's Mental Health
Katherine Ponte

Parents can and should play an active role in their college child's mental health in order to achieve the best possible college experience.

College is an exciting time for students and parents, but it can also be a critical time for your child's mental health. Here are a few suggestions on how you can help safeguard your child's mental health during this challenging and formative time.

Understanding mental health

Learn the basics about mental health conditions. The three most important concerns are depression, anxiety, and suicidal ideation — all are rising among college students. Seventy-five percent of all mental illnesses develop by age 24. There are many good online resources such as NAMI's website. Essentially, closely watch for any change in their behavior — are they withdrawing, are their reactions to stressors disproportionate to the stressful events they are experiencing, and is their emotional health adversely impacting their day-to-day functioning? Also bear in mind that substance use may exacerbate a mental health condition, and we know that exposure to alcohol and drugs may increase during these years and potential problems may develop. Encourage your child to reach out to their college counseling office for help if they are showing signs of emotional distress. Suicidal ideation and suicide have reached alarming rates and require immediate action. A few signs of suicide risk include expressions of hopelessness, talking about self-harm, and talking about unbearable pain or being a burden. Minority, first-generation, and international students may also be at greater risk due to particular stressors that these groups may encounter.

Talking about mental illness

Share what you've learn about mental health with your child. Talk about it. It can be very helpful to share your own college experiences with your child so that they feel you can relate. Emphasize to them that you'll always be there and support them. Let them know you may worry, but you'll worry more if they don't talk to you. Tell them it is common for college students to experience emotional distress and that they should not to be ashamed or embarrassed to talk about it if they have any concerns. Stay in touch with them as much as your child allows, especially when they are in distress. Most importantly, tell them if they ever experience thoughts of self-harm that they must immediately contact emergency resources, which includes their college's counseling office. Under HIPAA,_a counseling office must maintain the privacy of student treatment. Under FERPA, the counseling office may, but is not required to notify you of a serious mental health crisis or emergency. You should also urge them to call the National Suicide Prevention Hotline: 1.800.273.8255. Be firm.

On-campus resources

Know basic information before the school year start about on-campus mental health resources, including location, scheduling an appointment, drop-in service availability, after hour services, and access to peer support services. Learn if the college has wellness programs, which may offer self-care guidance and activities. Student mental health groups such as Active Minds (the leading college students' grassroots mental health organization), the Steve Fund (the leading college students' minority mental health organization), and The Jed Foundation (JED), the leading college mental health advisory and program development organization, may offer important support.

Stressors — a proactive approach

Stressors may trigger a mental health condition. The earlier potential stressors are identified, the sooner coping strategies may be applied to contain them. There are many stressors. The three key stressors for many students fall into three categories: loneliness, academic, and career. It is important to know possible stressors since your child may be more willing to discuss stressors than mental illness due to stigma. The Healthy Minds Network, the leading college student mental health academic research institute, is doing cutting-edge research in the area.

Resiliency

Resiliency is a valuable strength for combating the emotional impact of stressors. Resiliency is the ability to recover quickly from difficulties such as competitive environments, failure, setbacks, and disappointment.

Importantly, it can be bred and developed as we face these sorts of challenges. Tell your child that it may take a little while to adjust to college life as is true for many college students and that they can bounce back from initial challenges. Tell them that no matter what, you'll always be proud of them.

Loneliness

A majority of college students feel lonely. Let your child know how common it is. Encourage them to make new friends by participating in orientation activities, activities, and clubs. Again, stay in touch with them, especially during the first semester. Encourage them to call home. Suggest to them that they participate in self-care activities such as physical exercise, good nutrition, and athletics. Intramural sports is a great way to boost mental and physical health and connect with other students.

Academic performance

Academics is a key, and perhaps the greatest, source of stress for students. The high-school-to-college transition can be difficult. It is not uncommon to experience average-to-poor performance compared to high school, competition, imposter syndrome, perfectionism, and discouragement. Encourage your child to seek tutoring and to contact their college's accommodations and disabilities office, which may provide them with very helpful academic support, should they qualify. Help them develop academic related coping skills before starting college and throughout such as stress management, time management, and problem solving. Grades may be a strong indicator of possible academic struggle so it may be helpful for your child to share them with you — they can give you permission to access their grades under FERPA. Provide extra support, if required and possible. Finally, emphasize with them the critical importance of good sleep hygiene. Tell them these strategies will help them achieve better grades, which is the ultimate objective of many students.

However, if college stresses become overwhelming it may be best to consider taking a medical leave rather than dropping out as it may be more difficult to return in the latter case. A majority of college students who drop out of college do so for mental health reasons. There are many wonderful college re-entry programs to facilitate your child's return to college such as Fountain House's College Re-entry Program and others like it.

Career planning

Career planning can be a significant source of stress. It may start to intensify as your child considers internship opportunities. It could be highly beneficial to speak to a career office early on to explore options and understand hiring criteria such as course work, grades, work experience. You may also want to encourage your child to volunteer in an area of interest relevant to potential career goals, which may give them firsthand experience.

College can be an incredibly stressful time, but your help can be invaluable as your child transitions into adulthood. It is a time when your child can take more responsibility and ownership of their life decisions. But you can have a critical impact on their academic, career, and personal success by being an active participant and resource.

Originally published in *Thrive on Campus*, Jun. 30, 2019.

39

Taking a College Medical Leave
Katherine Ponte and Jason Bowman

College students across America are facing significant mental health challenges, leading some to call the situation a "campus mental health crisis". Many students are unaware and unprepared for these challenges. The social, academic, career planning, and financial pressures can all contribute to emotional stress. The high school to college transition alone can be challenging. There are ways to manage these challenges including effective coping strategies, professional treatment and accommodations. Yet, many students simply drop out when challenges become overwhelming and traditional alternatives fail. However, taking a medical leave may be the best short-term and long-term option. And fortunately, there are programs that can facilitate your return like Fountain House's College Re-entry Program.

Mental Health Challenges

According to the American College Health Association Fall 2019 National College Health Assessment, 27.6% and 21.5% of students experienced anxiety and depression, respectively, which can be overwhelming. A significant number of cases can worsen to a disorder when ongoing signs and symptoms cause frequent stress and compromise functioning. Co-occurring anxiety and depression disorders may make things even worse. Also, 50% of students experienced loneliness, which can lead to be isolation and withdrawal and be a risk factor for suicide, the second leading cause of death for college students. Indeed, college years are a critical time for mental illness development as 75% of all lifetime mental illness develops by age 24. College drinking rates are also high, which may also exacerbate a mental health condition. A mental health screening may help determine if professional care is appropriate.

Mental health problems and mental illnesses may be chronic, progressive, and/or debilitating, and they need immediate attention. They may impact physical health. They may also lead to relationship difficulties with friends and family, contributing to social isolation and withdrawal. The impact on academics may be significant. Mental health issues can affect a student's energy level, concentration, dependability, cognitive ability, and optimism, hindering performance. In fact, a student who is struggling with their mental health is twice as likely to leave college without graduating.

Medical Treatment on Campus

The initial step to addressing a mental health concern is to seek treatment at a college counseling office. However, on-campus mental health treatment may be limited. Counseling center utilization has significantly increased in recent years. Yet, most counseling centers are working with limited resources with fewer therapists than recommended.

Accommodations

Academic accommodations may be an effective option to help manage the academic impacts of mental health challenges. The most important accommodations for many students are extra time on exams and/or assignments. The *American with Disabilities Act* (ADA) and the Section 504 of the *Rehabilitation Act* ("Section 504") require college's to offer reasonable accommodations. Information may be found at the college's accommodations and disabilities office. Disclosure of a medical condition and documentation from a health care provider will be required.

Medical Leave

Where available mental health treatment and accommodations have failed to adequately address mental health concerns, a voluntary medical leave or leave of absence may be an effective option. A student's support team should be consulted, including the medical treatment team, family and academic advisors. During a leave, a student is not enrolled in classes, but intends to return. There are many potential benefits to taking a medical leave, but there are also important considerations. Above all, mental health should be prioritized.

Whether or not the leave is voluntary or involuntary, the ADA and Section 504 may afford a student with certain rights and protections. Students with mental health concerns engaged in self-injurious behavior may be placed on involuntary leave, which may be treated differently than a voluntary leave. It is important for students to carefully understand a college's policies, practices and procedures concerning a voluntary medical leave. The following are a few additional considerations for medical leave:

1. Academic – There are many academic issues to consider. These include the treatment of completed work and whether academic records will note an incomplete or withdrawal. These are important as they may impact future applications for graduate school, scholarships, internships, and employment. Confidentiality and privacy concerns should also be considered.

2. Financial – There may be many financial impacts if a student takes a leave, which should be carefully reviewed with university officials and public and private institutions granting scholarships and grants and lenders. Important considerations include:

    o Will amounts paid for tuition, housing, and meal plans be refunded or prorated? Is there an existing tuition insurance policy?

    o Will scholarships and grants be forfeited in part or in whole?

    o Will student loans be subject to early repayment?

   Inquiries on refunds, forfeitures, grace periods, accrual of interest, and deferments should be made. It may also be important to know if college health insurance will remain in effect. A college's Financial Aid Office or Bursar may offer guidance.

3. College privileges – It may be important to a student to maintain some form of connection with college friends. If allowed, continuation of student privileges such as access to college email accounts and student facilities may facilitate this.

4. Return to School - A return to school should be contemplated and planned. A few important considerations are documentation, deadlines, and conditions. A key issue is if re-application will be required. If a school places unreasonable. conditions on a return, a student may be able to file a grievance with the disability compliance officer.

While a voluntary medical leave may pose a number of challenges and risks, it may still be the best option. A few benefits, include:

1. Best care possible – Due to college counseling limitations, the best care possible may be available off-campus and under the

supervision of a familiar provider such as a former therapist or family doctor. This access may improve the chances of treatment compliance. Only 40% of students with mental illness seek help on-campus. Also, a strong support network, which may only be available at home, is important to overcoming mental health challenges.

2. Academic performance – Good mental health can maximize academic performance. Bad mental health may lead to significant disruptions in work, incompletes, dropped classes, lighter course loads, and lower GPAs. It may even place a student at risk for a mandatory leave due to poor academic performance. An involuntary leave may have more negative repercussions than a voluntary leave. Worse, poor academic performance may impact future academic pursuits, employment prospects and earning potential.

3. Social consequences – Social consequences are not as great as students may fear. During an absence a student may remain in touch with college friends. Good mental health may allow students to maintain better social relationships instead of the isolation and withdrawal so common when a person has mental illness. Many of these relationships are likely to continue even after a leave is taken and a student returns to college. In fact, at most public universities, only 19% of full-time students earn a bachelor's degree in four years.

In deciding whether to take a leave, the most important consideration must be mental well-being as it can impact every aspect of our lives now and in the future.

Fortunately, there are programs that can help a student return with significantly greater chances of better managing a mental health condition and excelling academically. Fountain House's innovative and groundbreaking College Re-entry Program is one such program.

Fountain House's College Re-entry Program

The College Re-Entry program's primary goal is to help students build self-confidence and develop the knowledge, skills, and abilities to succeed in school through academic, wellness, and social interventions. This, coupled with their ongoing, external clinical support, gives young adults the foundation they need to excel.

Participants

Through the College Re-Entry program, young adults ages 18-30 participate in a highly organized curriculum based on their unique needs. The program, which primarily serves students and families in the New York City tri-state area, focuses on engaging undergraduate college students who have withdrawn from their academic studies due to psychiatric disability (e.g. depression, anxiety, bipolar, and schizophrenia) by developing and implementing an action plan to return to college and providing the necessary skills and strategies to successfully reach their educational goals. The program is a non-clinical model working as a bridge between students' clinicians and colleges while a student is on leave. Through the COVID crisis, the program now offers a virtual curriculum allowing College Re-Entry to extend its reach.

Non-clinical Model

Attuned to the needs of young adults living with mental illness, and in the absence of a non-clinical approach addressing the growing needs of college students, Fountain House applied its community mental health model to develop the College Re-Entry program in 2014. Fountain House built the program based on the premise that it takes more than medication management and talk therapy to support a young adult student's successful return to college after a debilitating mental health interruption. It is within this vein that they built a comprehensive curriculum that:

1. Encompasses classes aimed at strengthening academic skills

2. Offers wellness workshops aimed at reducing stress and increasing resilience

3. Creates social opportunities aimed at combating social isolation and anxiety

Core Program

The Core program operates on a trimester schedule and offers a structured 14-week curriculum consisting of 15 hours of in-house classes per week,

1 hour of one-on-one coaching, and several additional social activities. After the completion of the Core program, College Re-Entry offers an additional semester of support for students who are back in school, ensuring a higher rate of college retention. Throughout the Core program and continued support semester, students are further supported by their academic coach who can help with all of the administrative details for returning to college. Alumni of the program can continue to get support from their coach as needed.

Academic Coaching

In addition to this curriculum, each student is paired with an academic coach who helps guide them through the process, as well as looks at their academic goals and logistics for re-entry. The College Re- Entry Center was built as a peer-supported space near Fountain House's main clubhouse to give young adults the opportunity to be around other college students who have had similar experiences. The College Re-Entry Center and the program itself mirrors a typical college environment and structure as much as possible, incorporating classes taught by college professors, along with spaces conducive to learning and socializing.

Impacting Student Lives

The College Re-Entry program has the capacity to dramatically change the lives of young adults living with mental illness. As a holistic early intervention program—the only one of its kind—College Re-Entry has been successful in keeping students engaged and getting them on the path to achieving their academic goals. In addition to helping 75% of students return to college, the program found statistically significant evidence showing that both self-efficacy and mental wellbeing improved for students after completing the program. Opportunity now lies in the expansion and replication of the College Re-Entry program on college campuses and in communities nationwide.

In the words of College Re-Entry Alumna Shannon Pagdon: "I was extremely fortunate with the group of people who went through the program with me; they all taught me a lot, and I am so appreciative of that. I also loved all the different subjects we covered, including notetaking, nutrition, budgeting, and self-care (and that is just a few things we covered!)."

The College Re-Entry program has been acknowledged as filling a critical need by educational partners, clinicians, and experts in the mental health field. Michael Birnbaum, M.D., Director of Early Treatment Program at North Shore, notes: "The early stages of mental illness interfere with precious periods of healthy development. Early intervention services, such as Fountain House's College Re-Entry Program, are designed to minimize disability, reduce symptoms, promote recovery, and instill hope. These interventions can have positive impact lasting a lifetime."

In Summary

More and more students are experiencing mental health challenges in college, but these are not insurmountable. There are on-campus resources and tools that can help such as counseling offices and academic accommodations. However, sometimes this help is not enough. Some students may require additional support that may not be available on campus. There are a number of alternatives to consider. For example, a medical leave can allow students the time and focus to treat and manage their illness and develop the self-care and academic coping strategies that will allow them to return to school better able to perform academically. Fortunately, there are programs like the Fountain House's College Re-entry Program that can help make this possible. They can help students pursue and achieve their dreams of earning a college education if threatened by mental illness. Unfortunately, many students simply do not know where to turn for help and what additional options may exist. Students who do not access available resources to address their mental health challenges may ultimately drop out. This outcome represents not only a personal loss, but a loss to society, that can be avoided.

Jason Bowman, Chief of Staff; Founding Director, College Re-Entry, Fountain House is a mission-driven non-profit leader with 20+ years of experience working in community mental health. As Fountain House Chief of Staff, he is charged with driving through strategic initiatives, facilitating organizational workflow and supporting the strategic vision of Fountain House CEO, Dr. Ashwin Vasan. As the Founding Director of College Re-Entry, he co-designed a program to help students with mental health challenges develop the knowledge, skills and abilities to re-enroll in college and succeed. Prior to that, he was the Director Fountain House Gallery, expanding it from a small volunteer program into the premier venue in New York City representing artists with mental illness. Jason earned a BA in Sociology from Marymount

167

Manhattan College and received his master's degree in public and nonprofit administration from Columbia University's School of International and Public Affairs.

References

American College Health Association, National College Health Assessment, 2018: https://adobe.ly/2OWAhZc
American College Health Association, National College Health Assessment, 2019: https://adobe.ly/2P0O94F
Bazelon, Campus Mental Health: Know Your Rights, 2008: https://adobe.ly/3jIv6KH
Healthy Minds, Investing in Student Mental Health, 2019: https://adobe.ly/3062SSq
The Jed Foundation: jedfoundation.org
National Alliance on Mental Illness, College Students Speak, A Survey Report on Mental Health, 2012: https://adobe.ly/303QaDy
National Council on Disability: ncd.gov
National Disability Institute: nationaldisabilityinstitute.org
Penn State, Center for Collegiate Health, 2017 Annual Report: https://adobe.ly/2EoB8js

Originally published in *Thrive on Campus*, July 27, 2020.

40
Mental Health Challenges in the LGBTQ+ Community
Rui Pires and Katherine Ponte

As a gay man, my earliest feelings of attraction to other men in adolescence were accompanied by an awareness that they conflicted with my immigrant parents' expectations. I suppressed outward displays of my sexual orientation and retreated. I grew depressed and anxious. I felt pressure not to upend my family's and society's expectations of me.

I ultimately found solace in a chosen family of friends in high school. They were mostly young women, also of minority and countercultures, who also did not conform to family expectations. Unfortunately, I was forced to leave them behind when I moved with my family to the town where I attended university. My new home offered no queer community or network of friends. My hope evaporated. And one day, I attempted suicide.

Sadly my story is not uncommon for someone in my community, as being LGBTQ puts a person at a higher risk for suicide attempts. LGB adults are also more than twice as likely as heterosexual adults to experience a mental health condition.

There are many reasons for this, including the discrimination, prejudice, violence and family rejection that people in the LGBTQ+ community experience. And while it is encouraging that in the last decade more communities are securing equal rights, non-discrimination protections and increasing public support for their civil and political rights, we still have a long way to go when it comes to LGBTQ+ mental health.

Here are some of the main challenges the community faces as well as suggestions for addressing them.

Coming Out and Family Estrangement

The rejection by family and close friends can be one of the most traumatic experiences for members of the LGBTQ+ community. Coming out is a very difficult process. According to a 2013 survey, Only 56% have told their mother, 39% have told their father, and 40% have experienced rejection from their family or a close friend.

When I finally came out to my parents, they concluded I must be sick. Surprisingly, the family doctor in our community rebuked them. His support helped me with anxiety and allowed my parents to tolerate my existence—although they seemed incapable of considering or prioritizing my well-being and happiness.

Substance Use and a Lack of Support

My university and early work years were a constant grind with little time for self-care and self-reflection. I escaped into short bouts of alcohol abuse and risky sexual behaviors. Substance use is an issue within the LGBTQ+ community. Research shows that 44% of LGB adults are likely to have problems with alcoholism compared to 24-33% for others.

I was also grappling with the stigma of HIV deaths in my new community. The proximity of death forced me to confront some basic questions about life. I was not coping well, and I couldn't rely on family for support or solace. So I had to seek support from a broader range of people.

Insufficient Health Care

LGBTQ+ mental health experiences are very individualized. Health needs of the LGBTQ+ community often are grouped together, yet each sub-community represents a distinct population with their own unique mental health challenges, rates of mental illness, experiences and coping strategies. We should address these issues accordingly. Additionally, knowing the appropriate language to describe gender identity and sexual orientation is important in understanding and recognizing this diversity.

Having a caring and understanding doctor can make a tremendous difference, but many people don't have access to this level of care. The key obstacles to effective mental health treatment are systemic harassment and lack of cultural competency, in addition to low rates of insurance coverage. As a result, 30% of LGB adults are more likely to delay or not seek medical care compared to 17% in other communities.

Those who receive treatment sometimes fear disclosing their sexual orientation or gender identity for fear of discrimination and gender bias. Therefore, doctors are often unaware of specific needs among LGBTQ+ patients, which may limit their ability to treat and advise them properly.

Suggestions for Improvement

There are many ways to improve mental health care, including early intervention, appropriate and comprehensive treatment and family support. It's important to recognize the challenges of coming out and the possible lack of family or chosen-family support. Health care providers must also address implicit bias and stereotyping.

There are also simple ways that health care providers can create a welcoming treatment environment. They can prominently display a non-discrimination policy and a pride or a trans-pride flag. Offering reading and informational material relevant to the community as well as knowing local LGBTQ+ resources helps. It also helps if employees avoid assumptions about gender identity and sexual orientation based on appearance and ask for one's preferred pronouns. They also should use gender-inclusive language on forms and while communicating with patients.

We need much more research on LGBTQ+ mental health needs. We could facilitate this research if the LGBTQ+ community were able to identify themselves fully on surveys. Eroding the barriers of stigma and rejection to coming out is key to addressing the additional risks these communities face. Additionally, members of the LGBTQ+ community identifying themselves enriches research on the community's mental health needs.

Everyone Deserves Effective Mental Health Care

After my third visit to an emergency room with severe exhausting chest pains, I realized that even after surviving a suicide attempt and facing the cumulative grief of the loss of many friends and clients due to HIV, I had to come to terms with the fact I had not made enough positive change in my life. I want to live fully, so I've been focusing much more on my own health and self-care. I've finally concluded that seeing a therapist would be beneficial. And with a few false starts, I am still hopeful I can find a good match for my own counseling needs.

Effectively addressing LGBTQ+ mental health disparities will require our society—including friends and family and medical providers—to affirm, accept and respect the LGBTQ+ community. Everybody deserves and is worthy of access to good mental health care and support to achieve the best outcomes, regardless of gender identity or sexual orientation.

Rui Pires has worked in queer sexual health for the past 30 years, with a simultaneous career in the community-based poverty field serving as a financial trustee with people who found themselves homeless due to chaotic substances use or due to severe mental health challenges. He has sat on the boards of directors of several non-profit social service, cultural and human rights groups. Rui has struggled with anxiety as a child and for all his adult life.

Originally published in *National Alliance on Mental Illness Blog*, Jul. 17, 2019.

41
Mental Health Challenges in Immigrant Communities
Katherine Ponte

My parents immigrated from Portugal to Canada, where I was born and raised in a large Portuguese immigrant community. I now have been living in the U.S. for 20 years.

The phenomenal work ethic of my community was a great source of pride. It inspired me to work as hard as I could, as my parents did. I became a lawyer and earned an MBA. My spouse is also of Portuguese descent and was born and raised in the U.S. His background reflects the same immigrant values and motivations.

My spouse and I were able to accomplish our goals, despite the fact that our parents came from very modest backgrounds. None of them graduated from high school or even spoke English at the time of their immigration. It is a common story, shared by so many immigrant children.

I was able to grasp the opportunities my parents worked so hard to provide. However, my quintessential hard-working immigrant success story still does not address a very important factor: I live with bipolar disorder. The mental health challenges that immigrants face are the part of this story that need to be addressed.

Immigrant Community Challenges

Immigrant communities encounter many challenges including discrimination, anti-immigrant sentiment and policy, language difficulties as many immigrants don't speak English upon their arrival, lower access to healthcare due to lower paying jobs without benefits and visa issues as some immigrants are undocumented, among many others. There is also the added challenge of isolation from the larger national community. Many immigrant families live within or very close to their immigrant community, which may reinforce a sense of separation.

Coping with these challenges can lead to mental health issues or mental illness, particularly for those with a pre-existing biological vulnerability to a mental illness.

Insufficient Mental Health Treatment

At the time of my parent's immigration, mental health education in their homeland was non-existent. There was rarely any discussion of mental health. When they arrived in Canada, they could not speak English. There were no Portuguese-speaking mental health care providers. And the few Portuguese-speaking doctors there had very heavy patient loads and did not address mental health during their short consultations.

In some immigrant communities, mental health concerns are actively ignored and people are discouraged from seeking help. Their reluctance is often out of fear that others might find out or due to high treatment costs. Some cultures also have alternative treatment approaches to mental health care such as herbal remedies or spiritual practices. For example, some communities use culturally rooted practices of mindfulness and meditations or religious practices such as prayer.

Stigma in the Community

In the Portuguese community where I grew up, mental illness was highly stigmatized. Women and men were reluctant to speak about it. If and when women expressed emotional concerns, they were quickly dismissed. Men never talked about emotional concerns since community perception was that strong men should not be emotional. Talking about mental health outside the home was prohibited. Family members also heavily gossiped in our close-knit community, causing people to be guarded or secretive.

Growing up, I never heard anyone in the Portuguese community talk about mental health, including my parents. I was shocked to be diagnosed with a mental illness many years later. Upon reflection, I think I showed signs of mental health issues as early as high school, but neither I nor my parents knew how to identify it, much less how to seek help. Parents can play an important role in the mental health literacy of their children, but often immigrant parents are not in a position to help.

Stereotypes

Common stereotypes of immigrants—that we are less educated, more blue-collar, more conservative—can adversely impact our mental health. To avoid these perceptions, we sometimes disassociate ourselves from our immigrant community. This may lead to a loss of network support, which is another risk factor for mental health issues.

Missing the Sense of Belonging

We may feel that we're not accepted here in the U.S., but in our parents' homes, we're also regarded as foreign or "American." So we don't have a clear identity of who we are. This can be troublesome for our mental health. The greatest sense of belonging I ever felt was with descendants of other Portuguese immigrants. A sense of belonging can be critical to good mental health, and at many times we lack it.

A Lack of Cultural Competency

As an adult, I have been treated by several doctors and therapists for my mental illness. I have never been asked about my cultural background by any of my therapists. When I have raised my cultural upbringing and experiences, they have been minimized, misunderstood and dismissed so many times that I don't even try to explain it anymore.

The challenges are even greater for those who cannot speak English. If and when they see a therapist, it can be incredibly difficult to express emotions in their non-native language. Translation can help, but a therapist might need stronger understanding for cultural context to really help a patient. Different dialects can also complicate translation. Many immigrants are far less likely to seek treatment or trust health care providers due to a lack of cultural understanding and competency.

Shortage of Mental Health Education for Faith Leaders

In the depths of my depression, I believed that God was angry at me, punishing me. It was at these times that my suicidal ideation was greatest. It would have really helped to speak to a faith leader who could have reassured me that I was wrong, but I didn't know who to turn to, as many faith leaders do not discuss mental health. I don't recall a single sermon in my many years of weekly Sunday masses that discussed mental illness. And some faith leaders, when presented with emotional concerns, guide their followers to prayer or to "pray it away."

Opportunities to Improve Mental Health

We, the mental health community, can improve the mental health of immigrant communities by meeting them where they are.

We can nurture relationships with faith leaders, who can play a tremendous role in immigrant mental health. Many people in immigrant communities turn to their faith leader first, before a health care provider when experiencing emotional distress. And houses of faith can be a great forum to spread information on mental health information and resources.

We can develop more informational campaigns in partnership with local community foreign language media. We could also make more foreign language mental health information available in places immigrants frequent, such as popular restaurants and social clubs.

We can encourage immigrants and their descendants to enter mental health professions and continue to encourage mental health professionals to prioritize cultural competency.

We can promote greater understanding and compassion of the unique challenges immigrants and their children face. It is indisputable that immigrants make tremendous contributions to our adopted country, and they—and their mental health—should be acknowledged, respected and valued.

Originally published in *National Alliance on Mental Illness Blog*, Jul. 22, 2019.

Part VI.
Rights and Advocacy

42

The Many Forms of Mental Illness Discrimination
Katherine Ponte

Discrimination against people with mental illness is widespread. It can be highly detrimental to reaching and staying in recovery. At times, as sad as it may be, the best way for us to manage discrimination is to know it exists, be prepared for it and know how to safeguard our rights.

People living with mental illness *should* have access to the same opportunities as everyone else. However, while protected by law, these rights are too often disregarded and regulations have fostered systemic discrimination. Our community often faces two layers of discrimination — the original act of discrimination and the discrimination we confront when trying to enforce our rights.

Despite these issues, pursuing your legal rights and protections is the most effective way to combat systemic discrimination and change laws. Here are a few examples of mental illness discrimination and ways to challenge unfair practices.

Health care — Cost Coverage

Medicaid and Medicare laws discriminate against people with mental illness. For example, one law prohibits federal Medicaid funding for non-elderly adults receiving psychiatric care in a treatment facility with more than 16 beds. No physical health conditions have this limitation. Medicare beneficiaries are also limited to 190 days of lifetime inpatient psychiatric hospital care. According to the National Association for Behavioral Healthcare, "No other Medicare specialty inpatient hospital service has this type of arbitrary cap on benefits." This is particularly harmful for people living with chronic serious mental illness (SMI) who often need more than 190 days of hospital care.

Refusal by health insurance companies to cover certain medications is another form of potential discrimination. However, you can appeal these refusals to legal and regulatory agencies. Some State Attorney General's Offices have a hotline for filing appeals.

Discriminatory regulations and laws can be the most difficult form of discrimination to challenge. To change laws, we need political advocacy and community action. You can take action on the local, state and federal levels. Join the advocacy efforts of your local NAMI affiliate and NAMI National, the Kennedy Forum, The Bazelon Center for Mental Health Law and Treatment Advocacy Center, among others.

Health care — Treatment

People living with SMI die an average of 25 years earlier than the general population. Most of us die from physical conditions and discrimination in the health care system may play a role. Evidence has shown that health care providers are liable to display negative attitudes and stereotyping behavior toward people with mental illness and incorrectly attribute physical symptoms to a person's mental illness.

One study found that health care providers who stigmatize were more likely to think patients with mental illness would not adhere to treatment and, therefore, less likely to refer them to a specialist or refill their prescriptions. Even some psychiatrists hold stigmatizing views against people with mental illness, which can significantly impact treatment outcomes.

Local and state mental health government offices can sometimes help in healthcare related discrimination. There may also be state-specific bodies that investigate complaints against doctors and other licensed professional.

Employment

Employment is the one of the most important factors for sustained mental health recovery. A literature review found that people with mental illness remain unemployed or underemployed at significantly higher levels compared to the general population. People with mental illness were shown to be perceived as incompetent and less promotable, receive lower wages and have less access to quality jobs. Even in terms of supporting existing employees with depression, about 25% of managers reported they did not feel confident in doing so effectively.

The American with Disabilities Act (ADA) and Rehabilitation Act of 1973 offer protections for job applicants and employees with mental illness. The ADA is enforced by several government agencies, notably the Equal Employment Opportunity Commission and the U.S. Department of

Justice. You can file a complaint with these agencies if you feel discriminated against on employment matters. You may also be able to file a complaint with your state's Fair Employment Practice Agency.

Housing

Access to adequate housing is another critical component of recovery in which people with mental illness may experience discrimination. Despite protections, people with mental illness tend to face discrimination when searching for housing according to a U.S. Department of Housing and Urban Development report. People with mental illness were less likely to receive:

- Responses to their inquiry about housing
- Notifications that an advertised unit was available
- Invitations to contact the housing provider or inspect the available unit

Many also received adverse treatment when asking for reasonable accommodations.

In cases of housing discrimination, you may be able to file a complaint under the Fair Housing Act. Local, state and federal levels often offer protections against housing discrimination.

Criminal Justice

People with mental illness experience higher rates of incarceration, disproportionate shares of prison populations and a lack of access to mental health treatment during incarceration. After being booked into jail, people with SMI stay 2-3 times longer in pretrial phase and face longer sentences. They are less likely to make parole and more likely to cycle through the system or die by suicide.

People with SMI housed in prisons and jails are three times the amount in hospitals. Yet, only one in three prison inmates receives any form of mental health treatment. Lack of care can worsen mental illness and lead to higher recidivism rates. A criminal conviction can severely limit access to resources needed to reach recovery. This is especially true for people with SMI who experience extremely high rates of co-occurring disorders.

Challenges include securing a job, housing assistance, educational financial aid and other government benefits.

Criminal matters are complex and appropriate legal representation may be critical. You may find a criminal lawyer in the Martindale Hubbell Legal Directory. State Bar Associations may be able to refer you to a legal services association that can offer low or free cost help. Another great source of assistance can be law schools, which sometimes have legal aid clinics where supervised law students provide guidance on legal matters. In some cases, it can be very beneficial to receive press coverage, but you must consider this option carefully.

Discrimination is an unpleasant reality for our community, but there are established ways and resources to combat it. It's essential to consider the risks and your chances of success before committing to legal action. However, advocating for your rights can be empowering and help you feel that you have some control over your life.

Each one of us must stand up to it to the best of our abilities. Action can benefit not only you, but all of us.

This article is for informational purposes only and does not constitute legal advice.

References

The American with Disabilities Act (ADA): https://www.ada.gov
Rehabilitation Act of 1973: https://bit.ly/2XmtqfD
Fair Employment Practice Agency: https://bit.ly/2LKhcYC
Fair Housing Act: https://bit.ly/3e8AGSO
Martindale Hubbell Legal Directory: https://www.martindale.com
State Bar Associations: https://bit.ly/3cVx1HO
Law Schools: https://www.nalplawschools.org

Originally published in *National Alliance on Mental Illness Blog*, Mar. 11, 2020.

43
Ways We Can Address
the Social Determinants of Mental Health
Katherine Ponte

Social determinants of health are "conditions in the places where people live, learn, work, and play [that] affect a wide range of health risks and outcomes." There are many, and they can affect both physical and mental health.

A focus on social determinants of health can lead to better mental health outcomes, including preventing mental illness. We all have a role to play in addressing them, individually and as members of society, working with local, state and federal government, nonprofits and companies.

Here are several examples of social determinants of health and potential ways to address them.

Economic Circumstances

Economic circumstances can significantly affect health risks and outcomes. Poverty, and particularly neighborhoods with a concentration of poverty, pose elevated health risks, including mental health disparities.

Creating economically integrated neighborhoods

As of 2014, almost 14 million people lived in extremely poor neighborhoods. The worst impacted were Hispanic and African American communities. They were more than three and nearly five times more likely, respectively, to live in an extremely poor neighborhood than poor whites.

People living in high-poverty neighborhoods exhibit worse mental health outcomes compared to people in low-poverty ones. Children can experience significant mental health problems from living in these environments, as can people with serious mental illness. This determinant is connected to reduced job opportunities, increased criminal activity and reduced quality of education in schools, which can contribute to other mental health stressors.

There are several initiatives that may address these challenges. One strategy is the creation of economically integrated neighborhoods. This concept can be accomplished in many ways, including the relocation of residents to less impoverished neighborhoods.

Increasing access to affordable housing

Poor housing can result in worse mental health. Adverse conditions such as dampness, mold and cold indoor temperatures may be associated with anxiety and depression. Worse yet, lack of affordable housing may lead to homelessness, which can exacerbate mental health issues. About 45% of the homeless population have mental illness.

A range of suitable housing programs should be available for those with mental illness. Access to affordable housing is certainly a larger social and governmental issue with meaningful implications for mental health. It is therefore an important area for advocacy.

Physical Environment

Certain physical settings, notably city environments, may pose greater risks to mental health. For example, the stimulation of an urban setting combined with a lack of green spaces and areas for exercise and social interaction can lead to sensory overload.

Dedicating spaces in cities for nature, exercise and socializing

There are four key areas that can improve mental health in urban settings:

1. More green spaces
2. Active spaces that encourage exercise
3. Social spaces that promote interaction
4. Safe spaces, free of crime and traffic

These environments can foster a sense of psychological security, which can positively affect mental health. Urban planning can play an important role in positively shaping social determinants of health. Therefore, these types of strategies must extend to impoverished communities where they are needed most.

Neighborhood Cohesiveness

A healthy community can be critical to good mental health. Community can provide a sense of belonging and a source of support, which both benefit mental health. Neighborhood cohesiveness is critical to fostering a positive community since it often determines a community's ability to act collectively on a wide range of issues, including mental health.

Many strategies can enhance cohesiveness, but here are two example that support community living and opportunities for recreational activities.

Build community gardens

Community gardens are collaborative projects in shared urban spaces. Participants share in the maintenance and products of the garden. In addition to being a source of food, community gardens create opportunities for people to work together to improve communities. The social interaction can reduce loneliness and social isolation, which are detrimental to mental health, in addition to many other benefits.

Establish community centers

In many neighborhoods, community centers serve "as a space for social interaction and the development of social relationships." Dedicated spaces for interaction, like community centers, can contribute to social capital, a sense of belonging and a sense of community. As a result, a community center can help participants feel empowered.

A community center, especially in a neighborhood with more limited services, should ideally offer a wide range of social interaction opportunities. Community centers can engage and support participants by offering:

- Age-appropriate activities for a wide range of age groups
- Specific programs for marginalized communities, respecting cultural diversity
- Whole health activities such as exercise and meditation
- Outdoor space
- Meeting places, like a coffee shop or eating area
- Health awareness education
- Assistance with government benefits and referral services

- Collaboration with outside organizations and professionals to offer services and supports

Volunteers can be recruited from within the community to help run programs. This engagement of community members may help build feelings of ownership, self-worth and purpose, all of which are beneficial to mental health.

Healthy Food Options

What you eat can significantly affect mental health. A growing body of evidence suggests that unhealthy eating patterns can lead to an increased risk for mental health conditions like depression and anxiety. An unhealthy diet can also lead to the development of various physical ailments, notably heart disease, stroke and type 2 diabetes, which in turn can worsen mental illness. For example, "people with diabetes are 2 to 3 times more likely to have depression than people without diabetes." The relationship between mental and physical health and the role diet can play are important considerations, as the life expectancy of adults living with serious mental illness is 25 years lower, on average, often due to chronic physical diseases.

Unfortunately, lower income communities are at a disadvantage in eating healthfully. Food deserts, which are neighborhoods or communities with limited access to affordable and nutritious food, are commonly found in urban, low-income areas. These communities are less likely to have nearby access to supermarkets or grocery stores with healthy food choices.

Bring healthy food options to underserved communities

There are a few ways to address this disparity. Nutrition and diet awareness in communities can help. More business-driven strategies include incentives for supermarkets to locate in underserved areas, incentives for bodegas and corner stores to offer more healthy choices and developing local farmers' markets.

Social inequities, reflecting decades-long systemic discrimination, have left impoverished communities at heightened risk for mental illness. To recognize and address these social inequities is to address the social determinants of health that disadvantage the mental health of these communities.

A significant and important segment of our population has been waiting too long for the government, companies and all of us to provide the equity they deserve.

Originally published in *National Alliance on Mental Illness Blog*, Aug. 7, 2020.

44
Mental Health Law Considerations, New York Example
Nawa Lodin, Esq.

Understanding mental health laws requires a vast understanding of several bodies of law that govern the treatment and rights of the patients. Families seeking to learn more about a patient's rights with regards to mental health should look to their state statutes, regulations, case law and guidance from their state mental health agencies. Many of these state regulations address three common themes: types of admissions to mental health facilities, court mandated assisted outpatient therapy and confidentiality. This article will address these themes with a focus on New York law.

Patients admitted to New York State psychiatric centers are admitted pursuant to New York State's Mental Hygiene Law. The New York state agency which regulates this law is the Office of Mental Health (OMH). Most states have dedicated agencies, typically within their department of health, that regulate and enforce their state mental health laws.

Admissions

Like many other states, there are three types of admissions in recognized under the New York Mental Hygiene Law: informal, voluntary and involuntary. Informal Admissions (9.15 MHL) is the least restrictive and allows for a patient to leave at any time. This level of admission requires that the patient be in need of treatment, request admission and be suitable for informal status. The patient can make an oral request for this type of admission with no written application (9.15). Voluntary admission, among other things, requires a patient to complete an application and the patient must notify the hospital in writing of their intention to leave the hospital. With the caveat that if the director of the hospital objects to the patient's release, that objection must be made within 72 hours for a court order of retention (9.13). Involuntary submissions are typically more complex and understandably include several requirements. An involuntary submission can be made by "medical certification" requiring two licensed physicians to submit the Office of Mental Health's standard form certifying that the patient meets the involuntary standard. The patient can be held involuntarily for up to 60 days (9.27). Another type of certification is that of a community services director or designated physician who certifies that the patient suffers from a mental illness severe enough to pose a risk to themselves or others. Involuntary admission can also be made by emergency admission. Emergency admission requires reasonable cause to believe a patient with mental illness for which immediate observation, care and treatment in a hospital is appropriate and which is likely to result in serious harm to him/ herself or others. Emergency admission is up to 15 days, unless the person has been converted to medical certification, or agreed to remain as a voluntary admission. New York is unique in that the New York Supreme Court has established an agency known as the Mental Hygiene Legal Service (MHLS). MHLS provides legal services and representations for patients and their families.

Kendra's Law

At least 48 states have some form of "assisted outpatient treatment" (AOT) laws. AOT is supervised treatment within a community, allowing for patients to remain in the community while still receiving treatment. In 1999, New York enacted legislation known as "Kendra's Law" for court-mandated AOT. The law was enacted as public safety measure after a series of incidents in which individuals suffering from mental illnesses became violent and caused serious harm to others. Originally proposed by members of the National Alliance on Mental Illness (NAMI) and other mental health organizations in New York, Kendra's Law granted civil courts the authority to order certain people to regularly undergo psychiatric treatment for a maximum for a 12-month period. Failure to comply can result in commitment for up to 72 hours. Referrals to AOT can be made by almost anyone with personal contact with the individual including friends, roommates and treatment providers. Among other factors, the criteria for requiring AOT includes (9.60): that an individual is "unlikely to survive safely in the community without supervision, based on a clinical determination" has a history of lack of compliance with treatment for mental illness that has resulted in acts of serious violent behavior toward self or others or threats of, or attempts at, serious physical harm to self or others within the last forty-eight months, not including any current period, or period ending within the last six months, in which the person was or is hospitalized or incarcerated. Supporters of Kendra's Law emphasize that it enables people with mental illness to maintain more of their civil liberties, rather than being ordered into a hospital. According to a 2005 study by NY OMH, recipients of AOT engaged in physical harm at 55% the rate of people with mental illness who do not receive AOT.

Confidentiality

The Health Insurance Portability and Accountability Act (HIPAA) limits the use and disclosure of protected health information (PHI). It does however allow for disclosure of PHI for treatment, payment and healthcare operations without patient authorization. It is worth noting one caveat- HIPAA provides greater protections and limits on disclosures of psychotherapy notes on the grounds that they are particularly sensitive. Nonetheless, in addition to federal regulations, one should also assess state laws on confidentiality and disclosure of mental health records.

Many states, including New York, have enacted regulations that require authorization to disclose mental health information. This additional authorization requirement in the case of mental health information is a stronger standard than HIPAA.

The NYS Mental Hygiene Law confidentiality requirements apply to clinical records that are created or maintained by a provider that is operated, licensed, or funded by OMH. This means that it would not apply to a private practitioner nor would they apply to a provider that is licensed by the NY Department of Health. Nevertheless, other laws, rules, or ethical standards might still apply to these types of providers.

Nawa Lodin is an attorney with Goodwin Procter, LLP. She focuses her practice on health care law and counsels clients on a wide variety of state and federal laws and regulations, particularly compliance with privacy laws, self-referral laws and reimbursement laws. Prior to joining Goodwin Procter she worked as assistant regulatory counsel for a national association which represents and advocates for ambulatory surgery centers.

45

A Primer on Government Benefits
Annie Harper, Ph.D.,
School of Medicine, Yale University

SSI and SSDI Benefits

People who struggle with their mental health to the extent that it affects their ability to work and earn a living, can apply for disability benefits from the Social Security Administration (SSA) to provide them with an income in lieu of employment income, or to supplement income from part-time work. There are two categories of public disability benefits. The first is Social Security Disability Income (SSDI), for people who have worked for a long enough period in the past to qualify through tax payments to Social Security. The second is Supplemental Security Income, which is available for people who have not worked long enough to qualify for SSDI. Many people receive a combination of SSDI and SSI; if the amount they get as SSDI is low, because of a limited work history, then it is supplemented by SSI to bring up to the standard SSI amount. Currently (as of 2020) while a person on SSDI can get a maximum of $3,011 monthly, the average monthly payment is around $1,200. The SSI maximum amount for an individual is $783 monthly (some states pay supplements). About 3.5 million people in the country receive SSDI and/or SSI because of a mental health disability.

When a person is receiving benefits, there are some important things they need to be aware of:

Income-earning and Asset Limits

This is probably the most important, and frustrating, aspect of living with disability benefits. There are strict, complicated rules on how much a person can earn and save, and unfortunately the benefits system does not do as good a job as it should of supporting people in understanding the rules, and in managing situations where their benefits may be affected. These rules can dissuade people from work; most people who receive SSDI and/or SSI do not become independent from those income sources, in part because of the complicated rules. It's important, if possible, to seek expert advice on such matters – there are some good websites out there (see resources below) and one-on-one counseling is available nationwide.

But, to get started, here are some key issues people should be aware of:

Asset Limits

- People getting SSDI only do NOT have to worry about asset limits. They can save as much money as they like, and own as many assets as they like, and their SSDI will not be affected.

- SSI recipients have to contend with much stricter asset limits. If a person on SSI has more than $2,000 at the beginning of the month, they are not eligible for SSI that month.

There are ways to avoid asset limits. Special needs trusts have long been an option for keeping money aside which does not trigger asset limits, but those trusts can have high fees, and can be complicated to administer, with the owner of the funds not allowed direct and unlimited access to the funds. Recently, a much more straightforward option has become available; ABLE accounts allow a person with a disability, diagnosed before the age of 26, to keep as much as $100,000 in assets without losing benefits. Advocates are pushing for the age restriction to be lifted. Also, the Pass program allows SSI recipients to save money for employment purposes through the Plan to Achieve Self-Support (PASS) program; any money saved is excluded from SSI asset limits.

Income-earning Limits

- SSDI recipients do have to pay attention to how much money they earn from work. The (very complicated) rule is that a person on SSDI can earn in addition to their SSDI, up to $910 every month (2020 numbers), and their SSDI is not affected in any way. However, if they earn up to what is known as the Substantial Gainful Activity (SGA), which in 2020 is $1,260, then they lose their SSDI entirely. If they earn more than $910 but less than $1,260, then they enter what is called a Trial Work Period; if they earn this amount for more than nine months within a 60-month period, then they lose their SSDI. Medicare coverage continues for 93 months after this. Yes, it is complicated!

- Income earning limits for people on SSI are easier to understand, but much more limiting. A person can earn, from work, up to $65 per month with no effect. After that, their SSI payment is reduced by 50 cents for every additional $1 they earn.

Managing overpayments

Given how complicated and confusing the rules about assets and income-earning limits are, it is extremely common for people on SSDI and/or SSI to be told by the SSA that they have got an 'overpayment' (continued to receive SSDI or SSI during a period when they were ineligible due to excessive assets or earned income) and have to repay the SSA. Recent research has found that 2/3 of people on SSDI who earn over the SGA for at least one month are overpaid at some point, with an average overpayment amount of nearly $10,000; the number is higher for those with a psychiatric disability. People who are told they have been overpaid and need to repay the SSA, can: appeal if they believe it is incorrect; ask for a waiver, if the overpayment wasn't their fault and repayment would cause hardship for them; or ask for a payment arrangement that they can manage.

These asset and income-earning rules are extremely complicated and confusing and can cause a great deal of financial and emotional stress for people. It's important that people try to educate themselves about the rules, but it's also important to understand that the current benefits system simply does not work well for people who it is supposed to help. People are often left blaming themselves for having gotten into a situation where they are now repaying the SSA, and struggling to pay their bills; we need to recognize that these situations, in the vast majority of cases, arise as a result of a broken and confusing system, not because of any individual failings.

Asset and income limits for other benefits

Though I won't go into detail about these here, many SSDI/SSI recipients may also be eligible for other benefits and subsidies, most notably Medicaid or Medicare, housing subsidies such as Section-8, and SNAP (food stamps). Those benefits may also be subject to asset and income-earning limits, which vary by state. See resources below to find information about SNAP asset limits in your state, Medicare asset limits, and Medicaid asset limits.

Debts

SSDI/SSI income is protected from many types of debts that people may owe, including credit card debt or medical bills; this is known as being judgement proof. However, there are some exemptions; people on SSDI (though not people on SSI) may have a portion of their income taken to repay certain government debts, such as back taxes, federal student loans, or child support.

Help managing money

Many, many people struggle to manage their money, regardless of whether they have mental health problems or not. We live in a world where it is getting harder and harder to cover basic expenses of life, where we are offered more and more opportunities to spend our money without thinking about it first, and where it is very easy to borrow money that we can't easily afford to repay. Four in ten people in America do not have $400 saved up in case of an emergency. People on SSDI/SSI, particularly those on SSI, have to manage on a very low income, which makes it even harder to stay on top of their finances.

- Giving someone else financial control: People who really feel that they cannot manage their money and keep getting into financial trouble, do have the option of handing financial control to another person. The two most common ways to do this are i) through giving financial control to a conservator of estate, who will manage all the person's financial affairs for them, or ii) through giving financial control to a representative payee, who will just manage any SSI/SSDI income the person gets. In this section I will just talk about representative payees (payee for short). While a person can choose to have a payee their money for them, it can also be required by the SSA, if they believe that an SSDI/SSI recipient is not managing their funds properly.

- Getting help but keeping control: Many people want some type of support managing their money, but do not want to hand control over to someone else. One option is to find a financial counselor or coach, if there is a local program that offers this service for free. Free services are available at financial empowerment centers (FEC). The Federal Trade Commission offers guidance on choosing a Credit Counselor.

- Making sure that banking works for you: Many people with disabilities do not have bank accounts, often because they feel they just don't have enough money, or they had an account in the past and ended up paying high fees, or because they get their money on a Direct Express card and don't see the need to have a bank account. If a person has a financial management system that works for them, there is no need to get a bank account. However, if they would rather have a bank account, there are things they can do to make sure that account works for them. Many banks now offer BankOn Accounts, which do not charge overdraft fees, and have no, or just a very low, predictable monthly fee. If a person would like to have someone keep an eye on their spending behavior, they can, with Wells Fargo bank, give another person 'view-only' privileges, which means that other person has a separate log-in and password to their account, and can look at online statements, but cannot touch the money in the account. People can also sign up for the Eversafe tool, which allows someone else to check on an account but not touch the money. Eversafe has a monthly charge, the lowest option is under $10. People can also ask their bank about setting text alerts or daily spending limits to help them manage their own spending behavior.

Advocacy for a better financial future for people with mental illness

As you can see from this chapter, while there are some crucial resources and support available to people with mental illness, there are some serious problems with the current benefits system, and with the options available to people to make the best of their financial situations. People are expected to live on far too little, particularly people on SSI; people who are disabled are much more likely than others to be poor, particularly people of color. Income-earning and asset limits are far too restrictive; if the amounts were indexed to inflation, they would be far higher than they are today. The bureaucratic hoops that people have to jump through are excessive and ridiculously complicated, and the Social Security Administration is so under-resourced that it often makes mistakes, and benefits recipients are left to deal with the consequences. It can get even more complicated when people also rely on other benefits and subsidies which may be affected by assets and income. The banking system currently does far too little to provide good financial services to people who are poor or people with mental illness. Efforts are underway around the country to change things – for more see the resources below.

Annie Harper has a Ph.D. from Yale University in cultural anthropology. She conducts research on how vulnerable populations, particularly low income people with mental illness, cope with poverty and financial difficulties, and how to support them in this area. She is particularly interested in understanding how the financial services and retail industries could better serve low income people generally, and people with mental illness in particular.

Resources

National Disability Institute: nationaldisabilityinstitute.org
AARP: aarp.org
Nolo: nolo.com
Disability Secrets: disabilitysecrets.com
SSA Redbook: ssa.gov/redbook/
Substantial Gainful Activity: https://bit.ly/3gpUYIH
ABLE Accounts: https://bit.ly/2VOY80W
Plan to Achieve Self-Support (PASS) program: https://bit.ly/2ZzndxX
SNAP Asset Limits: https://bit.ly/31KF4EE
Medicare asset limits: https://bit.ly/3iti3Ms
Medicaid asset limits: https://bit.ly/2Z33qIh
Financial Empowerment Centers (FEC): fecpublic.org
Federal Trade Commission, Choosing a Credit Counselor: https://bit.ly/31Jd9VH
BankOn Accounts: joinbankon.org
Eversafe tool: https://bit.ly/3iwEksI
Banking for All: Why Financial Institutions Need to Offer Supportive Banking Features: https://adobe.ly/2DafYVD

Appendix I.
Additional Resources

1

Collaborative Care Plan

Katherine Ponte and Izzy Gonçalves

Consumers, who live with a mental health condition, and loved ones working together using clear, supportive, and compassionate communication achieve better outcomes. The Collaborative Care Plan ("CCP") provides a framework for mental health consumers, their loved ones, and clinicians to better communicate. The goal is to facilitate shared decision-making by incorporating the expectations, needs, and roles of all participants. Balancing the sometimes conflicting needs of the consumer and their loved ones is a sound foundation for long term recovery. Using the CCP, the consumer's care network together develops treatment objectives, responsibilities, and action plans. Developing a CCP when participants have clarity of mind without the pressures of an unfolding crisis can help mitigate and manage the everyday challenges and extreme uncertainty associated with mental illness. The biggest uncertainty may well be how we will be impacted and behave in a mental health crisis. Moreover, the CCP can make both the consumer and their loved ones feel better about the treatment process as they all have a say and sense of ownership in the process. This dynamic may foster a virtuous cycle of improved interpersonal relations, decreased symptomology, increased consumer compliance, improved self-care, and reduced caregiver fatigue.

I. Principles

Of the three principal parties in collaborative care, the consumer, the family or other loved ones, and the clinician, it is most often the consumer who is reluctant to participate and early to terminate. Therefore, actions that engage the consumer and keep them engaged are to be emphasized and pursued. The design and implementation of the CCP may be guided by these principles, which may also guide treatment relationships generally. It is important to acknowledge and appreciate that there is no one-size-fits-all approach to treatment. Treatment approaches must be open-ended and flexible to easily adapt to varying circumstances. They should be revisited often to recognize the evolving nature of a mental illness.

The following principles seek to maximize consumer engagement in the collaborative care process.

Principle 1: Improved Consumer Outcomes

Consumer outcomes improve if the consumer accepts family involvement in care and families are amicably involved in care.

Principle 2: Consumer-Family-Clinician Alliance is Critical

No fault is attributed to any of these parties for the mental illness.

Principle 3: Consumer-Driven Care

Consumer responsibility, ownership, and self-empowerment enhance consumer engagement. To maximize consumer engagement, care is consumer-driven. The family and clinician play critical supporting roles. Each party contributes equally, but, in normal course, deference is typically granted to the consumer's preferences and objectives unless their judgment has been substantially impaired. When a consumer is provided more control over the process, they are more likely to continue treatment and be more agreeable to family participation in care.

Principle 4: Shared Decision-Making

Shared decision-making that helps consumers achieve their self-determined life goals can empower consumers and encourage them to take ownership and responsibility for their care. As such, clinicians shall share their expertise with patients, provide them with available options, and allow them to choose their preferred course of treatment. Clinicians should support consumers in their decision, except in cases of impaired capacity.

Principle 5: Impaired Capacity

Consumers, families, and clinicians should all acknowledge the reality that certain severe mental health conditions can impair someone's capacity to fully understand the nature of their condition and exercise reasonable judgment about their treatment preference. Dialogue about that possibility and its potential forms and outcomes should be encouraged before an emergency situation and potential necessity for involuntary treatment.

Principle 6: Mutual Respect

Consumers, families, and clinicians have mutual respect for each other's experiences, preferences, and objectives. Experiences living with a condition, supporting someone with a condition, and treating someone with a condition are each respected and considered relevant to informing someone's care, particularly when these views are integrated. Establishing clear and transparent agreed upon methods of communication between consumers, families and clinicians builds and enhances trust.

Principle 7: Consumer Illness Objective

The illness is the object of the care, not the family. Treatment should be recovery-oriented and wellness targeted. In family therapy, the family itself is the object of treatment.

Principle 8: Strengths not Deficits Based

Emphasize the strengths of the CCP participants as opposed to deficiencies. Respective contributions should be acknowledged and respected.

Principle 9: Education and Resources using Evidence-Based Practices and Emerging Best Practices

Consumers and families benefit when they are educated about mental illnesses and have access to appropriate resources. The clinician should be actively engaged in assisting and guiding this. Evidence-based and emerging best practices should guide treatment decisions.

Principle 10: Ongoing Guidance and Skills Training

Clinicians provide consumers and families ongoing guidance and skills training, especially crisis management, enabling them to better manage the illness.

Principle 11: Well Delineated Uncomplicated Problem-Solving

Approach

Preventative approaches to problem solving are always preferred and sought. Using a structured, but flexible, problem solving approach helps consumers, families, and clinicians define and address issues. It is beneficial to break down complicated issues into small, manageable steps that they more easily address.

Principle 12: Validation and Emotional Support of All Parties

Experiences and feelings of each party are validated. Social and emotional support lets consumers and families know that they are not alone. Such a setting allows for open discussion and problem-solving.

II.   Instructions

1. Consumer completes all applicable sections first.

2. Caregiver completes next, agreeing to carefully consider consumer's entries.

3. Consumer and caregiver discuss together.

4. Consumer, caregiver, and clinician meet to finalize plan.

We should always strive to use "person first" language, meaning that the consumer is not defined by their condition. An example of "person first" framing would be "person is living with a diagnosis of bipolar" not a "person is bipolar". This CCP uses the term consumer to refer to a person living with a diagnosis of a mental health condition, instead of patient. Patient implies a medical setting, and often connotes a passive role in relation to the "doctor."

1. Objectives

Consider not only direct mental health condition management, but also the eight dimensions of wellness.*

What is Important to Consumer?

What is Important to Caregiver?

What is Important to Clinician?

Similarities Among What Three Parties Want

Differences Among What Three Parties Want

2. Key Treatment Details and Responsibilities

Care team

Party	Contact Information
Consumer	
Clinician	
Caregiver	
Other	

Diagnosis (clinician)

Treatment Responsibilities

Item	Who and What		
Medication			
Therapy			
Other			

Medication(s)

Name	Dose	Time(s) to Take

Therapy

Date	Who Attends	Agenda

Self-care (e.g. grooming, house chores, meals, exercise, meditation, etc.)

Item	Describe (including schedule)

3. Consumer Triggers / Early Warning Signs that Consumer May Need Help		
Trigger / Early Warning Sign	Who Responds (clinician, caregiver, consumer)	Response / Coping Strategy(ies)

4. Relationship Sensitivities regarding Mental Health Condition

These sensitivities can substantially impact the consumer's mental health, relationships, and consumer's receptiveness to a collaborative care approach. Complete the below statements:

Consumer to Caregiver: You make me feel better when...

Consumer to Caregiver: You make me feel worse when... (including triggers, concerns)

Consumer to Clinician: You make me feel better when...

Consumer to Clinician: You make me feel worse when…(including triggers, concerns)

Caregiver to Consumer: You make me feel better when…

Caregiver to Consumer: You make me feel worse when… (including triggers, concerns)

Caregiver to Clinician: You make me feel better when...

Caregiver to Clinician: You make me feel worse when... (including concerns)

Clinician to Consumer: You make me feel better when...

Clinician to Consumer: You make me feel worse when…(including concerns)

Clinician to Caregiver: You make me feel better when…

Clinician to Caregiver: You make me feel worse when…(including concerns)

5. Responsibilities and Results

Establishing responsibilities and intended results takes away some of the uncertainty of mental health management, which can be a significant source of stress. Consumers, caregivers, and clinicians shall use their best efforts to keep their reasonable responsibilities, but it also recognized that this will not always be possible. Where the behavior is unreasonably repeated, there shall be no discussion, and certain actions should result. Where any party is unable to keep their responsibility, the matter will be carefully reviewed and discussed. Good results shall result from good behavior, and bad results shall result from bad behavior. Often the focus of mental health treatment is on bad behavior with little or no recognition of good behavior. Recognition and rewards for good behavior should encourage consumers to remain healthy.

Consumer to Caregiver and Clinician

Time Frame (indicate daily, weekly, monthly)	Responsibility I will...	Intended Result (what: impact on consumer, caregiver, clinician)

215

Time Frame (indicate daily, weekly, monthly)	Responsibility I will...	Intended Result (what: impact on consumer, caregiver, clinician)

Consumer to Caregiver and Clinician

Time Frame (indicate daily, weekly, monthly)	Responsibility I will not...	Intended Result (what: impact on consumer, caregiver, clinician)

Caregiver to Consumer and Clinician

Time Frame (indicate daily, weekly, monthly)	Responsibility I will...	Intended Result (what: impact on consumer, caregiver, clinician)

Caregiver to Consumer and Clinician

Time Frame (indicate daily, weekly, monthly)	Responsibility I will not...	Intended Result (what: impact on consumer, caregiver, clinician)

Clinician to Consumer and Caregiver

Time Frame (indicate daily, weekly, monthly)	Responsibility I will...	Intended Result (what: impact on consumer, caregiver, clinician)

Clinician to Consumer and Caregiver

Time Frame (indicate daily, weekly, monthly)	Responsibility I will not....	Intended Result (what: impact on consumer, caregiver, clinician)

6. Notification of Concern

Consumer to Caregiver

Notify by *(in-person, call, text, email)*	Concern / Include Clinician?				

Caregiver to Consumer

Notify by (in-person, call, text, email)	Concern / Include Clinician?				

7. Planned Discussions

Parties	Time	Topic

8. Conflict Resolution

Gravity (minor, moderate, serious)	Issue(s)	Parties in Conflict	Final Decision

9. Incapacitation

Clinician decides

Description

10. Crisis Preparation

The application of the Collaborative Care Plan may significantly reduce crises, but we should always be prepared to address a crisis. Crisis preparation allows a consumer to feel more control and comfort, provided that their previously articulated treatment preferences are respected. Taking these measures in advance also positions family members to better manage a crisis. The best approach is to complete a Psychiatric Advance Directive ("PAD") (http://www.nrc-pad.org/). The PAD includes a statement of your treatment preferences, including where you wish to receive treatment (home, hospital outpatient, hospital inpatient), treatment you prefer to receive, treatment you do not wish to receive, including medication and other arrangements while ill. The PAD should include specific provisions concerning those the consumer may care for such as a child, spouse, etc. If you are unable to complete a PAD, it may still be helpful to have this discussion with your caregiver and clinician.

Eight Dimensions of Wellness

Making the Eight Dimensions of Wellness, developed by Peggy Swarbrick, part of daily life can improve mental and physical health for people with mental and/or substance use disorders.

What is Wellness?

Wellness is being in good physical and mental health. Because mental health and physical health are linked, problems in one area can impact the other. At the same time, improving your physical health can also benefit your mental health, and vice versa. It is important to make healthy choices for both your physical and mental well-being.

Remember that wellness is not the absence of illness or stress. You can still strive for wellness even if you are experiencing these challenges in your life.

What Are the Eight Dimensions of Wellness?

Learning about the Eight Dimensions of Wellness can help you choose how to make wellness a part of your everyday life. Wellness strategies are practical ways to start developing healthy habits that can have a positive impact on your physical and mental health.

The Eight Dimensions of Wellness are:

1. Emotional—Coping effectively with life and creating satisfying relationships

2. Environmental—Good health by occupying pleasant, stimulating environments that support well-being

3. Financial—Satisfaction with current and future financial situations

4. Intellectual—Recognizing creative abilities and finding ways to expand knowledge and skills

5. Occupational—Personal satisfaction and enrichment from one's work

6. Physical—Recognizing the need for physical activity, healthy foods, and sleep

7. Social—Developing a sense of connection, belonging, and a well-developed support system

8. Spiritual—Expanding a sense of purpose and meaning in life

You can access a copy of this document online at:
https://www.forlikeminds.com/collaborative_care_plan
To obtain a copy of this document in Microsoft Word,
please contact us at: hello@forlikeminds.com

2
The Transtheoretical Model (Stages of Change)

The Transtheoretical Model (also called the Stages of Change Model), developed by Prochaska and DiClemente in the late 1970s, evolved through studies examining the experiences of smokers who quit on their own with those requiring further treatment to understand why some people were capable of quitting on their own. It was determined that people quit smoking if they were ready to do so. Thus, the Transtheoretical Model (TTM) focuses on the decision-making of the individual and is a model of intentional change. The TTM operates on the assumption that people do not change behaviors quickly and decisively. Rather, change in behavior, especially habitual behavior, occurs continuously through a cyclical process. The TTM is not a theory but a model; different behavioral theories and constructs can be applied to various stages of the model where they may be most effective.

The TTM posits that individuals move through six stages of change: precontemplation, contemplation, preparation, action, maintenance, and termination. Termination was not part of the original model and is less often used in application of stages of change for health-related behaviors. For each stage of change, different intervention strategies are most effective at moving the person to the next stage of change and subsequently through the model to maintenance, the ideal stage of behavior.

1. Precontemplation - In this stage, people do not intend to take action in the foreseeable future (defined as within the next 6 months). People are often unaware that their behavior is problematic or produces negative consequences. People in this stage often underestimate the pros of changing behavior and place too much emphasis on the cons of changing behavior.

2. Contemplation - In this stage, people are intending to start the healthy behavior in the foreseeable future (defined as within the next 6 months). People recognize that their behavior may be problematic, and a more thoughtful and practical consideration of the pros and cons of changing the behavior takes place, with equal emphasis placed on both. Even with this recognition, people may still feel ambivalent toward changing their behavior.

3. Preparation (Determination) - In this stage, people are ready to take action within the next 30 days. People start to take small steps toward the behavior change, and they believe changing their behavior can lead to a healthier life.

4. Action - In this stage, people have recently changed their behavior (defined as within the last 6 months) and intend to keep moving forward with that behavior change. People may exhibit this by modifying their problem behavior or acquiring new healthy behaviors.

5. Maintenance - In this stage, people have sustained their behavior change for a while (defined as more than 6 months) and intend to maintain the behavior change going forward. People in this stage work to prevent relapse to earlier stages.

6. Termination - In this stage, people have no desire to return to their unhealthy behaviors and are sure they will not relapse. Since this is rarely reached, and people tend to stay in the maintenance stage, this stage is often not considered in health promotion programs.

To progress through the stages of change, people apply cognitive, affective, and evaluative processes. Ten processes of change have been identified with some processes being more relevant to a specific stage of change than other processes. These processes result in strategies that help people make and maintain change.

1. Consciousness Raising - Increasing awareness about the healthy behavior.

2. Dramatic Relief - Emotional arousal about the health behavior, whether positive or negative arousal.

3. Self-Reevaluation - Self reappraisal to realize the healthy behavior is part of who they want to be.

4. Environmental Reevaluation - Social reappraisal to realize how their unhealthy behavior affects others.

5. Social Liberation - Environmental opportunities that exist to show society is supportive of the healthy behavior.

6. Self-Liberation - Commitment to change behavior based on the

belief that achievement of the healthy behavior is possible.

7. Helping Relationships - Finding supportive relationships that encourage the desired change.

8. Counter-Conditioning - Substituting healthy behaviors and thoughts for unhealthy behaviors and thoughts.

9. Reinforcement Management - Rewarding the positive behavior and reducing the rewards that come from negative behavior.

10. Stimulus Control - Re-engineering the environment to have reminders and cues that support and encourage the healthy behavior and remove those that encourage the unhealthy behavior.

Source

Boston University School of Health: https://bit.ly/3gbnRc1

3
Active Listening

The active listening skillset involves these 6 active listening skills:

1. Paying attention

2. Withholding judgment

3. Reflecting

4. Clarifying

5. Summarizing

6. Sharing

These skills are discussed in more detail below. Several examples are used to illustrate the skill, in several case using the coach / coachee framework.

1. Pay attention

One goal of active listening and being an effective listener is to set a comfortable tone that gives your coachee an opportunity to think and speak. Allow "wait time" before responding. Don't cut coaches off, finish their sentences, or start formulating your answer before they've finished. Pay attention to your body language as well as your frame of mind. Be focused on the moment, and operate from a place of respect as the listener.

2. Withhold judgment

Active listening requires an open mind. As a listener and a leader, be open to new ideas, new perspectives, and new possibilities when practicing active listening. Even when good listeners have strong views, they suspend judgment, hold any criticisms, and avoid arguing or selling their point right away.

3. Reflect

When you're the listener, don't assume that you understand your coachee correctly — or that they know you've heard them. Mirror your coachee's information and emotions by periodically paraphrasing key points. Reflecting is an active listening technique that indicates that you and your counterpart are on the same page. See below examples:

Example 1: Your coachee might tell you, "Emma is so loyal and supportive of her people — they'd walk through fire for her. But no matter how much I push, her team keeps missing deadlines." To paraphrase, you could say, "So Emma's people skills are great, but accountability is a problem."

Example 2: If you hear, "I don't know what else to do!" or "I'm tired of bailing the team out at the last minute," try helping your coachee label his or her feelings by saying something like: "Sounds like you're feeling pretty frustrated and stuck."

4. Clarify

Don't be shy to ask questions about any issue that is ambiguous or unclear. As the listener, if you have doubt or confusion about what your coachee has said, say something like, "Let me see if I'm clear. Are you talking about …?" or "Wait a minute. I didn't follow you."

Open-ended, clarifying, and probing questions are important active listening tools that encourage the coachee to do the work of self-reflection and problem solving, rather than justifying or defending a position, or trying to guess the "right answer."

Examples include: "What do you think about …?" or "Tell me about …?" and "Will you further explain/describe …?"

The emphasis is on asking rather than telling. It invites a thoughtful response and maintains a spirit of collaboration.

Using Example 1 above, you might say: "What are some of the specific things you've tried?" or "Have you asked the team what their main concerns are?" or "Does Emma agree that there are performance problems?" and "How certain are you that you have the full picture of what's going on?"

5. Summarize

Restating key themes as the conversation proceeds confirms and solidifies your grasp of the other person's point of view. It also helps both parties to be clear on mutual responsibilities and follow-up. Briefly summarize what you have understood while practicing active listening, and ask the other person to do the same.

Using Example 1 again, giving a brief restatement of core themes raised by the coachee might sound like: "Let me summarize to check my understanding. Emma was promoted to manager and her team loves her. But you don't believe she holds them accountable, so mistakes are accepted and keep happening. You've tried everything you can think of and there's no apparent impact. Did I get that right?"

Restating key themes helps both parties to be clear on mutual responsibilities and follow-up.

6. Share

Active listening is first about understanding the other person, then about being understood as the listener. As you gain a clearer understanding of the other person's perspective, you can begin to introduce your ideas, feelings, and suggestions. You might talk about a similar experience you had or share an idea that was triggered by a comment made previously in the conversation.

Once the situation has been talked through in this way, both you and your coachee have a good picture of where things stand. From this point, the conversation can shift into problem solving. *What hasn't been tried? What don't we know? What new approaches could be taken?*

As the coach, continue to query, guide, and offer, but don't dictate a solution. Your coachee will feel more confident and eager if they think through the options and own the solution.

How to Improve Your Active Listening Skills

Many people take their listening skills for granted. We often assume it's clear that we're listening and that others know they are being heard. But the reality is that we as leaders often struggle with tasks and roles that directly relate to active listening. Accepting criticism well, dealing with people's feelings, and trying to understand what others think all require strong active listening skills.

Even with the best of intentions, you may actually be unconsciously sending signals that you aren't listening at all.

You may need to brush up on your listening skills if any of the following questions describe you. Do you sometimes:

- Have a hard time concentrating on what is being said?

- Think about what to say next, rather than about what the speaker is saying?

- Dislike it when someone questions your ideas or actions?

- Give advice too soon and suggest solutions to problems before the other person has fully explained his or her perspective?

- Tell people not to feel the way they do?

- Talk significantly more than the other person talks?

If you answered *yes* to any of these questions, you're not alone. To boost your active listening skills and put your active listening skillset into practice, try these helpful tips:

1. Limit distractions. Silence any technology and move away from distractions so that you can pay full attention to the other person. Take note of the person's tone of voice and body language as well.

2. Pay attention to what is being said, not what you want to say. Set a goal of being able to repeat the last sentence the other person says. This keeps your attention on each statement.

3. Be okay with silence. You don't have to always reply or have a comment. A break in dialogue can give you a chance to collect your thoughts.

4. Encourage the other person to offer ideas and solutions before you give yours. Aim to do 80% of the listening and 20% of the talking.

5. Restate the key points you heard and ask whether they are accurate. "Let me see whether I heard you correctly…" is an easy way to clarify any confusion.

Being a strong, attentive listener will help you be a strong leader as well. Your co-workers and direct reports will respect you more, and you'll likely see improvements in your relationships with them as a result. If you work to develop your active listening skills, you will not only become known as a good listener, you will become a better leader as well.

Source

Center for Creative Leadership: https://bit.ly/2Eafxev

4
Reframing

To reframe, step back from what is being said and done and consider the frame, or "lens" through which this reality is being created. Understand the unspoken assumptions, including beliefs that are being used.

Then consider alternative lenses, effectively saying "Let's look at it another way".

Challenge the beliefs or other aspects of the frame. Stand in another frame and describe what you see. Change attributes of the frame to reverse meaning. Select and ignore aspects of words, actions and frame to emphasize and downplay various elements. Examples include reframing:

- A problem as an opportunity
- A weakness as a strength
- An impossibility as a distant possibility
- A distant possibility as a near possibility
- Oppression ("against me") as neutral ('doesn't care about me")
- Unkindness as lack of understanding

The following examples apply some of these reframing techniques to statements:

- "It can't be done in time. But what if we staged delivery or got in extra help? I'm sure we can produce an acceptable product in the timeframe."
- "It does seem stupid, but it's also stupid not to look again and see what else can be done."
- "It's not so much doing away with old ways as building a new and exciting future."

You can often change a person's frame simply by changing their emotional state, making them happier, more aggressive, etc. When they are happier, for example, they will be more positive and optimistic (and vice versa).

Source

Changing Minds: https://bit.ly/32IbmAP

5
SMART Goals

SMART is an acronym that you can use to guide your goal settings. Goals should be:

1. Specific (simple, sensible, significant).

2. Measurable (meaningful, motivating).

3. Achievable (agreed, attainable).

4. Relevant (reasonable, realistic and resourced, results-based).

5. Time bound (time-based, time limited, time/cost limited, timely, time sensitive).

See below for more detailed discussion of these criteria:

1. Specific

   Your goal should be clear and specific, otherwise you won't be able to focus your efforts or feel truly motivated to achieve it.

   A specific goal may address questions such as:

   - What do I want to accomplish?

   - Why is this goal important?

   - Who is involved?

   - Where is it located?

   - Which resources or limits are involved?

2. Measurable

   Measurable goals allow you to track your progress and stay motivated. Assessing progress helps you to stay focused, meet your deadlines, and feel the excitement of getting closer to achieving your goal.

   A measurable goal should address questions such as:

   - How much?

   - How many?

- How will I know when it is accomplished?

3. Achievable

   Your goal also needs to be realistic and attainable to be successful. In other words, it should stretch your abilities but still remain possible.

   An achievable goal will usually answer questions such as:

   - How can I accomplish this goal?

   - How realistic is the goal, based on other constraints, such as financial factors?

4. Relevant

   This step is about ensuring that your goal matters to you, and that it also aligns with other relevant goals. We all need support and assistance in achieve our goals, but it's important to retain control over them.

   A relevant goal can answer "yes" to these questions:

   - Does this seem worthwhile?

   - Is this the right time?

   - Does this match out other efforts/needs?

   - Am I the right person to reach this goal?

5. Time-bound

   Every goal needs a target date, so that you have a deadline to focus on and something to work toward. This goal helps to prevent everyday tasks from taking priority over your longer-term goals.

   A time-bound goal will usually answer these questions:

   - When?

   - What can I do six months from now?

   - What can I do six weeks from now?

   - What can I do today?

Using the SMART goals approach will help you more easily set goals, stay on track towards achieving them and actually achieve what you really want.

Source

Adapted from Mind Tools - https://bit.ly/2ZSmBoy

6
Mental Health Education

Academy of Peer Specialist Services
https://www.academyofpeerservices.org/

Applied Suicide Intervention Skills Training (ASIST)
https://www.livingworks.net/

Boston University Center for Psychiatric Rehabilitation Book Store
https://cpr.bu.edu/store-info/

Coming Out Proud Program: Honest, Open, Proud
https://bit.ly/3gNWYLT

Emotional CPR
https://www.emotional-cpr.org/

Guide for Faith Leaders
https://adobe.ly/2XX4taD

Illness Self-Management Tool - CPI — Wellness Self-Management
WSM and WSM+ Workbook
https://practiceinnovations.org/Products

Illness Self-Management Tool - Enhanced Illness Management and
Recovery Manual
https://adobe.ly/3gS83vy

Illness Self-Management Tool - Honest, Open, Proud Program
http://www.comingoutproudprogram.org/

Illness Self-Management Tool - Pathways to Recovery
Purchase at Amazon: https://amzn.to/3O1NK8Z

Illness Self-Management Tool - Psychiatric Advance Directives (PADS)
https://www.nrc-pad.org/

Illness Self-Management Tool - Recovery Library
https://recoverylibrary.com/

Illness Self-Management Tool - Recovery Workbook I & II
https://bit.ly/3gTf9zE

Illness Self-Management Tool – WRAP
https://bit.ly/2MtF9E1

Intentional Peer Support
https://www.intentionalpeersupport.org/

Mental Health First Aid
https://www.mentalhealthfirstaid.org/

NAMI Find Course Locations - https://bit.ly/2AA7V3a

NAMI Basics – for caregivers of children and adolescents
https://bit.ly/2XVIdhn

NAMI Ending the Silence – 50-presentation for young adults
https://bit.ly/2MqGKuf

NAMI Family-to-Family – for caregivers
https://bit.ly/3dqCvL0

NAMI Homefront – for friends and caregivers of military service members
https://bit.ly/300fECe

NAMI Hope for Recovery – for adults living with mental illness

NAMI In Our Own Voice – trained speakers sharing their story
https://bit.ly/3dqHAD7

NAMI Peer-to-Peer – for people living with mental illness
https://bit.ly/3dx1tIy

Psychiatric Rehabilitation and Recovery Academy
https://www.psychrehabassociation.org/academy

Recovery Library
https://recoverylibrary.com/

Relias Academy – individual courses
https://reliasacademy.com/rls/store/

Rutgers Department of Psychiatric Rehabilitation and Counseling Professions
https://shp.rutgers.edu/

SBIRT – Addiction Screening, Brief Intervention, Referral to Treatment
https://sbirt.clinicalencounters.com/

Self-Assessment - Hope
https://adobe.ly/2Y1JEuI

Self-Assessment – Loneliness
https://adobe.ly/309fnNh

Self-Assessment - Internalized Stigma
https://adobe.ly/304eyVX

Self-Assessment - Social Support
https://adobe.ly/2MnrZbE

Self-Assessment - Quality of Life
https://adobe.ly/2U7KWmM

Self-Assessment – Recovery
https://adobe.ly/3eMj0N9

Serious Mental Illness Advisor
https://smiadviser.org/

Substance Abuse and Mental Health Services Administration (SAMHSA)
https://www.samhsa.gov/

Temple University's College of Public Health's Department of Rehabilitation Sciences
https://bit.ly/2Xvi763

Temple University Collaborative on Community Inclusion
http://www.tucollaborative.org/

Wellness, 8 dimensions of wellness
https://cspnj.org/resources/

WRAP – Wellness Recovery Action Plan
https://mentalhealthrecovery.com/wrap-is/

7
Mental Health Non-profits

National Alliance on Mental Illness
National Alliance on Mental Illness-New York City
National Alliance on Mental Illness Local Affiliates nami.org/findsupport

Active Minds
American Foundation for Suicide Prevention
Anxiety and Depression Association of American
Bazelon Center for Mental Health Law
Black Emotional and Mental Health Collective
Bring Change 2 Mind
Buddy Project
Child Mind Institute
Compassionate Friends
Crisis Text Line
Depressed Black Gay Men
Depression and Bipolar Support Alliance
Eating Disorders Information Network
Faces and Voices of Recovery
Fountain House
Gateway to Post Traumatic Stress Disorder Information
Heads Up Guys
Healthy Minds Network
iFred
International Bipolar Foundation
International OCD Foundation
Intrusive Thoughts
Jed Foundation
The Kennedy Forum
Letters Against Depression
Live Through This
Many Therapy
Mental Health America
Mental Health Channel
Mental Health First Aid
Mental Health Government

Military with PTSD
Mood Disorders Support Group
Mood Network
NADD
National Council for Behavioral Health
The National Eating Disorders Association
National Federation of Families for Children's Mental Health
National Institute of Mental Health
National Resource Center for Hispanic Mental Health
National Suicide Prevention Lifeline
Now Matters Now
Objective Zero
PFLAG - Parents, Families, and Friends of Lesbians and Gays
Project Health
Project UROK
Project Semicolon
SAMHSA – Substance Abuse and Mental Health Services Administration
Schizophrenia and Related Disorders Alliance of America
Shatterproof
Speaking of Suicide
The Stability Network
Stigma Fighters
Stop Soldier Suicide
Suicide Awareness Voices of Education
This is My Brave
ThriveNYC
Thunderbird Partnership Foundation
The Treatment Advocacy Center
The Trevor Project
Ulifeline
Warm Lines
Wounded Warrior Project
And many more
Canada
Anxiety Disorders Association of Canada
Bell Let's Talk
Canada Drug Rehab Addiction Services Directory
Canadian Association for Suicide Prevention

Canadian Mental Health Association
Centre for Suicide Prevention
Crisis Services Canada
Defeat Depression
Depression Hurts
Family Association for Mental Health Everywhere (FAME)
First Nations and Intuit Hope for Wellness Help Line
Gerstein Crisis Center
Good 2 Talk
Healthy Minds Canada
Kids Help Prone
Mental Health Commission of Canada
Mind Your Mind
Mood Disorders Society of Canada
National Eating Disorder Information Centre
National Network for Mental Health
Schizophrenia Society of Canada
And many more
See here for website links: https://bit.ly/2Y1NQKW

8
Suicide Prevention Resources

National Suicide Prevention Line
nationalsuicidepreventionlifeline.org
1-800-273-8255

American Foundation for Suicide Prevention
afsp.org

Crisis Text Line
crisistextline.org
text HOME to 741741 (24/7

The Trevor Project
thetrevorproject.org
866-488-7386 (24/7), Text START to 678678

The Veterans Crisis Line
veteranscrisisline.net
800-273-8255 and press 1 (24/7), Text 838255 (24/7)

Vets4Warriors
vets4warriors.com

SAMSHA's National Helpline (substance abuse)
samsha.gov/find-help/national-helpline
800-662-HELP (4357) (24/7) |

The National Alliance on Mental Illness
https://bit.ly/3fblmFS

The Jed Foundation
jedfoundation.org

Speaking of Suicide
speakingofsuicide.com

CDC Suicide Resources
cdc.gov/violenceprevention/suicide/resources.html

9
Peer Supporters/Peer Specialists

Career Description

Peer Support Provider Defined by iNAPS (International Association of Peer Supporters)

"Peer support providers are people with a personal experience of recovery from mental health, substance use, or trauma conditions who receive specialized training and supervision to guide and support others who are experiencing similar mental health, substance use or trauma issues toward increased wellness.

The term peer supporter is an umbrella for many different peer support titles and roles, such as peer advocate, peer counselor, peer coach, peer mentor, peer educator, peer support group leader, peer wellness coach, recovery coach, recovery support specialist, and many more....

In general, a peer supporter is an individual who has made a personal commitment to his or her own recovery, has maintained that recovery over a period of time, has taken special training to work with others, and is willing to share what he or she has learned about recovery in an inspirational way.

In many states, there is an official certification process (training and test) to become a qualified "peer specialist." Not all states certify peer support providers, but most organizations require peer support providers (who are employed) need to complete training that is specific to the expected responsibilities of the job (or volunteer work). Often, a peer supporter has extra incentive to stay well because he or she is a role model for others.

Those who provide authentic peer support believe in recovery and work to promote the values that: recovery is a choice, is unique to the individual, and is a journey, not a destination. Also, self-directed recovery is possible for everyone, with or without professional help (including the help of peer specialists or peer providers)."

See: Part III. Treatment Recovery, 24: Mental Health Peer Specialist Support

Useful Information

iNAPS National Practice Guidelines for Peer Supporters
https://adobe.ly/3cvLOYS

SAMHSA's Working Definition of Recovery
https://adobe.ly/3cUb2ku

Exploring the Value of Peer Support
https://bit.ly/3dwvqbW

Integrating Peer-support Services
https://bit.ly/3gSDk19

SAMHSA Peer Providers
https://bit.ly/2MtwUaR

Qualifications

State-by-state requirements

htttps://adobe.ly/3gKIdJT

Basic qualifications, include: personal experience living with mental illness, a high school diploma (GED), currently in recovery (stable, well) from mental illness, completion of state approved educational requirements, completion of ongoing state approved educational requirements, completion of state approved work experience, issuance of formal state certification.

Peer Specialists may also work under other job titles such as Peer Support Worker, Peer Support Specialist, Recovery Coach, Peer Navigator, Peer Bridger, Recovery Guide among other job titles.

Dual Certification – Mental Illness and Substance Use

Many people living with mental illness also have a co-occurring substance use condition — as high as 65%. If may be beneficial to obtain both mental illness and substance use recovery coaching certifications. Each State has their own Substance Use Certifications.

Addiction Counselors
https://www.addiction-counselors.com/

National Certified Peer Recovery Support Specialist (NCPRSS)
https://www.naadac.org/certification

Alternative Lived Experience Careers

Social Worker

As an alternative to being a peer support specialist, of all the professions you can directly apply your lived experience, becoming a social worker seems to be the most popular option.

National Association of Social Workers

U.S. News Best Social Work Programs

Certified Psychiatric Rehabilitation Practitioner

Psychiatric Rehabilitation Association

Marriage and Family Therapist

American Association for Marriage and Family Therapy

Lawyer

American Bar Association

U.S. News Best Law Schools

Licensed Professional Counselors

American Counseling Association

Occupational Therapist

The American Occupational Therapy Association

U.S. News Best Occupational Therapy Programs

Pastoral Counselor

American Association of Pastoral Counseling

Psychiatric Nurse Practitioner

American Psychiatric Nurses Association

U.S. News Best Nursing Programs

Psychiatry

American Psychiatric Association

U.S. News Best Medical Schools: Psychiatry

U.S. News Best Medical Schools

Psychologist

American Psychological Association

U.S. News Best Graduate Psychology Programs

10
Additional References in Chapters

Trustworthy sources for mental illness information and resources:

National Alliance on Mental Illness: https://nami.org/

Mayo Clinic: https://www.mayoclinic.org/

Key references for chapters in this book are listed at the end of each chapter. The below references provide additional support for data and statements made within chapters.

Chapter 5

Two Antidotes to Stigma

https://bit.ly/2QT4aL0

https://bit.ly/32WQX9r

https://bit.ly/3h5Geil

https://bit.ly/31U5T94

https://bit.ly/3hXjIcH

https://bit.ly/2EMNjar

Chapter 6

Embracing the Diversity Within Us

https://bit.ly/31Y7efb

https://bbc.in/3gX2rPw

https://bit.ly/32SWHkE

https://mayocl.in/2QOV5mu

https://bit.ly/2Dw6gxo

https://bit.ly/3gRYStK

https://bit.ly/352m71Q

https://adobe.ly/2Z5hPTC

https://bit.ly/3jITnzf

https://adobe.ly/3bp7bMw

Chapter 9

Talking About Mental Illness: Reaching In

https://bit.ly/3gYNb4m

https://bit.ly/31VNXuG

https://bit.ly/2Z54wmp

https://bit.ly/3gZBXg9

https://bit.ly/3539d3L

https://adobe.ly/2GurFrV

https://bit.ly/3gZC6QJ

https://bit.ly/3lNCPrR

https://bit.ly/2Z2ONEa

https://bit.ly/32QcroA

Chapter 18

Finding the Best Medication Regimen

https://bit.ly/3e4IDbV

https://bit.ly/2zTH15I

https://bit.ly/3h0M5oO

https://bit.ly/3bImjTT

https://bit.ly/32SXxxO

https://bit.ly/3lHYotM

https://bit.ly/2DsNw1D

https://bit.ly/354yZEI

https://bit.ly/3lHYy4m

https://bit.ly/3bnmwgG

https://bit.ly/32WuaL1

https://bit.ly/32SXxxO

https://bit.ly/3boA0IQ

Chapter 22

People With Mental Illness Can Work

https://bit.ly/2GsMTq6

https://bit.ly/31WS3D5

https://bit.ly/3lNDQQH

https://bit.ly/356T65c

https://adobe.ly/2GtAlid

https://bit.ly/2zcT0eS

https://bit.ly/2DqefMe

https://bbc.in/31YJlUV

https://bit.ly/3hlAyBK

https://bit.ly/2zcVaes

https://bit.ly/2Z5ke0A

https://bit.ly/2DsEMIZ

https://bit.ly/32ZDNJ7

https://bit.ly/3gSDk19

Chapter 23

The Mental Health Movement in the Workplace

https://bit.ly/2AMu5Px

https://bit.ly/31UkZLW

https://bit.ly/3gUCiRb

https://bit.ly/3btUgsS

Chapter 25

Building Mental Health Resilience

https://mayocl.in/2QUVB2o

https://bit.ly/3g76OYL

https://bit.ly/32WKhIE

https://bit.ly/3bq99fv

https://bit.ly/3boBrac

https://bit.ly/2Z5lnVW

https://bit.ly/32V42Af

https://bit.ly/3hSZEIe

https://bit.ly/353dwvP

https://bit.ly/355kEYU

https://bit.ly/32UAD9s

https://bit.ly/31WTO39

https://nyti.ms/2z0hCap

https://bit.ly/2Z4FUdb

Chapter 26

Ways to Manage and Cope with Stress

https://bit.ly/3i14djN

https://bit.ly/2R6htbf

https://bit.ly/3h5KzC9

https://bit.ly/2Z7lbp8

https://bit.ly/32SUhmg

https://bit.ly/2R6hEmV

https://bit.ly/355aC9R

https://bit.ly/3gX6njg

https://adobe.ly/3jOJqAB

https://mayocl.in/353KZGI

https://bit.ly/2R6hQTb

https://bit.ly/31ULikY

https://bit.ly/3gYQVmq

https://go.nature.com/2QUWI24

https://mayocl.in/3bof7xH

https://bit.ly/31ULikY

https://adobe.ly/2Z51QVK

https://bit.ly/2EZwHw7

https://bit.ly/2Z48bRj

Chapter 27

The Remarkable Human Animal Bond

https://bit.ly/2Z6I7Vs

https://bit.ly/2Z8YkJV

https://bit.ly/3buEI7S

https://bit.ly/3lS4nwk

https://bit.ly/3lTfGEg

https://adobe.ly/3jHgrOQ

https://bit.ly/3bpa1Be

https://bit.ly/3azFqQX

https://bit.ly/2Dtf8ni

https://bit.ly/3btQiQT

https://adobe.ly/2GuQXWS

https://bit.ly/3h01BRR

https://bit.ly/3i0ARlG

https://bit.ly/3kKf2st

https://bit.ly/32WRcSb

https://bit.ly/32V3yu1

https://bit.ly/3h02Dxt

https://bit.ly/2QXwk7H

https://bit.ly/3e8AGSO

https://bit.ly/32YWCvH

https://nyti.ms/3lTD30v

https://bit.ly/330zJbc

https://bit.ly/32UZwSs

https://bit.ly/31Z1W39

https://nyti.ms/3i0l0DH

https://bit.ly/2Z9rska

https://bit.ly/334dul4

https://bit.ly/2QWfoOU

https://bit.ly/2QR472m

https://bit.ly/3jSdrzz

https://bit.ly/3jZ7n8v

https://bit.ly/2QUJbHF

https://bit.ly/2QVMNta

https://bit.ly/3i3mhKi

https://bit.ly/2QYHI2U

https://bit.ly/2QVN0MY

https://bit.ly/3322WTe

https://bit.ly/320rYmx

https://bit.ly/3gZivQJ

https://bit.ly/2Dtr7Bi

Chapter 33

Suicide: Saving Lives Now and Beyond

https://bit.ly/31Y4YV4

https://bit.ly/3jPjiFQ

https://bit.ly/3jMHQzc

https://bit.ly/3lQBm45

https://bit.ly/2EPfRjz

https://bit.ly/356Xd12

https://bit.ly/3i3leKb

https://bit.ly/3bpEq2m

https://bit.ly/3i6h84c

https://bit.ly/2QVpHmi

https://bit.ly/3lNalyq

https://bit.ly/3bsnacz

https://bit.ly/3jMHQzc

https://bit.ly/31PqdZj

https://bit.ly/31Z3Xwj

https://bit.ly/2F5mjCC

https://nyti.ms/32StAxW

https://bit.ly/320ZbOR

https://bit.ly/2EXvMME

https://bit.ly/2GoHaBu

https://adobe.ly/356PobK

https://bit.ly/31Zc3VF

https://adobe.ly/3lTN65J

Chapter 35

Preventing and Preparing for a Mental Health Crisis

https://bit.ly/3h0lQiz

https://bit.ly/3gZYYQ7

https://bit.ly/321642G

https://adobe.ly/332cAoU

https://nyti.ms/2XviJZC

https://bit.ly/3bu3FR4

https://bit.ly/330RKWS

https://bit.ly/3jNOXr6

https://bit.ly/3i1p8mG

https://bit.ly/3i1pauO

https://bit.ly/3lQ6vVh

https://bit.ly/2F2Meem

https://to.pbs.org/357NhEG

Chapter 37

Suicide Prevention for College Students

https://bit.ly/3brJfbn

https://bit.ly/31ZnLzB

https://bit.ly/2Z9LDOW

https://bit.ly/3bsCt53

https://bit.ly/3gUt8UQ

https://bit.ly/3jNAlI9

https://bit.ly/2EYY2yr

https://bit.ly/3i3pSI0

https://bit.ly/3i1kVzF

https://bit.ly/2Z2jNnV

Chapter 38

What do Parents Need to Know About Their College Child's Mental Health?

https://adobe.ly/2QXqFP2

https://bit.ly/2Gzeiqx

https://bit.ly/3jJ8s43

https://adobe.ly/2EScSXE

https://bit.ly/35ah4wr

https://bit.ly/2F3Gxg4

https://bit.ly/3bv5lcQ

https://bit.ly/3h0pB7p

https://bit.ly/2EXfl2M

https://amzn.to/2F21F6C

https://amzn.to/3gY5CX1

https://bit.ly/3i3pSI0

https://bit.ly/3i1kVzF

https://bit.ly/2Z8mR1F

https://bit.ly/2F2M1YD

https://bit.ly/2F3Gxg4

https://bit.ly/33dc1ZN

https://bit.ly/2Z7z9HT

https://bit.ly/2Z6Qel4

https://amzn.to/2QUJ52N

https://adobe.ly/2EScSXE

https://bit.ly/2QUDjOz

https://bit.ly/2GvexTo

https://bit.ly/2CtR8Q8

https://bit.ly/3i1kVzF

https://bit.ly/3563Y3l

https://bit.ly/2QSkvQd

Chapter 39

Taking a College Medical Leave

https://adobe.ly/2F7T7uE

https://adobe.ly/3buhOh9

https://adobe.ly/2QTDN7w

https://adobe.ly/2OWAhZc

https://bit.ly/3gUt8UQ

https://bit.ly/3bqKirY

https://bit.ly/31ZYUM8

https://bit.ly/3brJfbn

https://bit.ly/3lOdj5H

https://bit.ly/2Z9LDOW

https://bit.ly/31WQm8E

https://bit.ly/3lQRMJL

https://bit.ly/3jJ8s43

https://adobe.ly/2Z5m9lQ

https://bit.ly/2DvFuoT

https://bit.ly/2CtR8Q8

https://adobe.ly/2EXjJyM

https://adobe.ly/2EXjQuc

https://adobe.ly/3583EkK

Chapter 40

Mental Health Challenges in the LGBTQ+ Community

https://bit.ly/2Z2pGBx
https://pewrsr.ch/331rHPB
https://adobe.ly/31YmxEu

Chapter 41

Mental Health Challenges in Immigrant Communities

https://adobe.ly/352zRK9

Chapter 42

The Many Forms of Mental Illness Discrimination

https://adobe.ly/3gXlSaD
https://bit.ly/3bq9jUn
https://bit.ly/3lZ4xCf
https://bit.ly/2QVMyhv
https://bit.ly/3hVykZU
https://bit.ly/2Gx2Tr9
https://bit.ly/32Vw6Ud
https://bit.ly/3hYOfXm
https://bit.ly/32WQX9r

https://bit.ly/2QUIoGD

https://on.ny.gov/3lOyxjX

https://bit.ly/3gSoZ3I

https://bit.ly/2QVILkm

https://bit.ly/2Duno6y

https://bit.ly/2XmtqfD

https://bit.ly/3h0w4zt

https://bit.ly/2LKhcYC

https://bit.ly/2CIA75o

https://bit.ly/3hBCW6Y

https://bit.ly/333dbZ0

https://bit.ly/3e8AGSO

https://bit.ly/3jO9yM0

https://adobe.ly/3bER0uR

https://adobe.ly/2Z7JXpi

https://bit.ly/31ZYgy8

https://bit.ly/2Z7b2ZI

https://bit.ly/3jQMegD

https://bit.ly/2QVpb7N

https://bit.ly/3cVx1HO

https://bit.ly/3bv2KzD

Chapter 43

Ways We Can Address the Social Determinants of Mental Health

https://bit.ly/3hZvDGV

https://brook.gs/31ZppkE

https://bit.ly/2GmlK83

https://bit.ly/3buu6WO

https://bit.ly/3h1Wq3O

https://bit.ly/32125mB

https://bit.ly/3h7fsWQ

https://bit.ly/2Z7UOzH

https://bit.ly/2Z9pwIt

https://bit.ly/3i18C6m

https://bit.ly/35cxQv7

https://bit.ly/2Z5thyw

https://bit.ly/2QSG1nX

https://bit.ly/3lRmUJ1

https://bit.ly/352QipP

https://bit.ly/2QUpNe3

https://bit.ly/3i0cd4L

https://bit.ly/2F6Mhpv

https://bit.ly/2Z3OA3C

https://bit.ly/3lN51eB

https://bit.ly/3bs0lpy

https://bit.ly/32RJB76

https://bit.ly/32T2mqY

https://wb.md/3lT7qEf

https://bit.ly/3h2ubCd

https://bit.ly/32XRyrB

https://bit.ly/3gZYYQ7

Appendix II.
ForLikeMinds

1
ForLikeMinds Explained

Our founder was diagnosed with bipolar I disorder over 15 years ago. Her spouse has supported her through extreme ups and downs. ForLikeMinds is born out of our personal recovery experience. It is dedicated to the recovery and wellness of people affected by mental illness, substance use, or stressful life events.

An astounding 1 in 5 Americans experience mental illness every year, and millions more are impacted by it in the United States alone. We know that overcoming stigma is a key first step towards mental health recovery and wellness. The light of hope illuminates the path away from the shadows of stigma towards recovery.

ForLikeMinds empowers members to connect and communicate one-on-one and in groups to support, inform, and inspire each other's recovery journey. This journey starts with hope and is nourished by the support of like minds sharing their lived experience. We would like to use this inaugural newsletter to introduce ForLikeMinds.

Awareness is improving but we're only starting to address unmet needs

Mental health awareness is increasing, which is very positive. This evolution is evidenced by the proliferation of apps and web-based services focused on mental health in recent years. These offerings vary in scope, target market, and functionality. We have only scratched the surface of potential benefits to mental health perceptions, treatment, and management from improved education and delivery tools.

ForLikeMinds seeks to address these yet unmet needs and untapped potential. We are different from existing online mental health tools in many important ways. Our approach is innovative and highly attuned to the experiences and needs of those affected by conditions and stressful events. It is rooted in our unique appreciation for the power of shared experience.

Focus on mental health conditions

Several websites allow users to connect with people across all types of medical conditions. We think mental health should have its own community platform given its medical and personal complexities and the sheer magnitude of people who experience a mental health issue every year. We think addressing mental health requires unique insight and functionalities. We are the only online community with a recovery- and wellness-oriented mission for people with a mental health or substance use condition.

Stigma is a stifling and heavy weight for people affected by mental health issues. At ForLikeMinds, you connect anonymously with relatable micro-communities of others like you, overcoming the fear and paralysis wrought by stigma. The process is intuitive and user-friendly. The platform offers many tools to control your experience on the site, particularly the quality and relevance of connections you make.

We recognize that mental health conditions often co-occur with substance use issues. The relationship between mental health and substance use conditions is particularly strong. ForLikeMinds is the only online mental health platform for those affected by either or both types of conditions.

We also recognize that so many stressful life events impact and trigger conditions. In many cases, you cannot separate discussing mental health issues from certain events and experiences. Comorbidity is also very common as many people with mental health or substance use issues also have or develop chronic health conditions. Engaging with others that have had similar experiences can be valuable in addressing mental health. ForLikeMinds facilitates connections based on a wide array of stressful life events and chronic health conditions that are often interconnected with mental illness and substance use.

A place for supporters too

We are the first dedicated mental health platform to serve interests of both people living with or supporting someone with a condition. No other online destination is tailored specifically to the needs of supporters. We embrace and acknowledge the important role supporters play in the recovery and well-being of their loved ones. We allow supporters to find and engage with other supporters to also realize benefits of peer-based support.

Focus on shared lived experience with people who can relate

Our founder is a rare example of a mental health entrepreneur who is actually living with a diagnosed mental health condition. When she started taking ownership of her condition, she researched alternative approaches to managing mental health. She found and immersed herself in peer support. This is a kind of grassroots approach to managing mental health. Sharing experiences and learning from others with like experiences can be very instructive, supportive, and inspirational. She concluded that peer support had tremendous untapped potential to help so many people beyond her.

You are not defined by a mental health condition. We recognize that mental health needs to be viewed and approached in the context of your personal background. Our unique circumstances impact illness onset, treatment, management, and recovery. Our mental health naturally impacts who we are and our relationships. Unlike other offerings, our approach focuses on addressing individual mental health needs through individual and group connections and engagement.

Member control and flexibility

ForLikeMinds is a platform for and by its members. We focus on acceptance and inclusion and recognize that different communities have unique mental health needs. When researching existing peer-based online mental health tools, our founder had a difficult time finding forum discussions or stories with which she could relate directly. Most platforms focus on facilitating groups or forums that are fairly generic, typically based on a common condition, like depression or anxiety. They lack tools to find or form connections based on more specific conditions and individual backgrounds.

Our user-friendly approach allows members to easily connect one-on-one and in groups based on a wide range of shared characteristics. We call them "Tags". You select Tags in your profile to search for matching groups and members or to identify groups you create. These Tags include age, location, gender identity, sexual orientation, ethnicity and race, language, religion, education, profession, student status, and military status.

This approach allows our members to find groups and members with experiences that are relevant and relatable to your own — someone with a condition or a supporter, the specific condition, stressful life event, personal and cultural backgrounds. We allow anyone to create and lead a group and give them powers normally reserved to an administrator. We think of these groups as micro-communities defined by their Tags. In addition to being thought leaders, Group Leaders have the power to remove posts and members to enhance the group experience. We have heard some tell us that people with mental illness should not be allowed to lead their own groups on our platform. We disagree, but focus on providing a welcoming environment with user tools to manage the quality of their experience.

A place for communities with unique mental health issues

Cultural and societal differences can significantly influence whether or not we seek help, what type of help we seek, what coping styles and support we have, and what treatments might work for us. Some communities experience higher rates of mental illness, higher rates of stigma, lower rates of treatment, and poorer access to resources. These include the LGBTQ+, military, student, and certain ethnic communities. Even when able to access treatment, these communities often receive poorer quality care due to lack of cultural competence, bias, and inadequate resources.

ForLikeMinds is for these unique groups. Much of our community outreach has also focused on facilitating peer support within these unique communities. Members of the military community can connect based on service period, branch, deployment, and combat history, and any exposure to military sexual trauma. We are the only online mental health platform that allows students to connect based on their university. College life is exciting, but also very challenging. It is a critical period for mental health. More than 75% of all mental health conditions begin before the age of 24. It is common for students to feel stressed and overwhelmed. A rising number of students are also struggling with sexual assault on campus and self-injury. Student suicide rates have reached alarming highs. A peer-to-peer community can help address the unique mental health needs of this population.

Only the beginning

Recovery is a long and complex journey. There is much more we hope to offer over time. We believe our unique insights and ongoing engagement with you will allow us to address your unmet needs. Please help us tap the potential of our community and shared experiences.

As part of the platform, we will have an informative blog and newsletter. We will also seek to collaborate and create partnerships with others who share our mission, including individuals and organizations.

Launched October, 2018

Visit ForLikeMinds: ForLikeMinds.com

Watch our How to Video: https://bit.ly/2LOEFYF

Share our Flyers:

General - https://adobe.ly/3gUnovH

Caregivers - https://adobe.ly/3dDE8Fm

2
Video Script: A Recovery Journey
Katherine Ponte

Hello, my name is Katherine Ponte. I have bipolar disorder, and I'm in recovery. Recovery in mental illness is living a full and meaningful life. Most don't believe recovery is possible for the mentally ill, not even the mentally ill themselves. I don't recall many "get well soons". And there were no flowers on my psych ward.

Bipolar struck me down as I entered the prime of my life. Triggered by several stressful life events, I was first diagnosed with depression then bipolar disorder over 15 years ago while in graduate school. I spent years refusing treatment, denying my condition which held me hostage. I cycled up through severe mania and down to major depression for too many years. While I resisted my diagnosis, I could not deny the consequences. I was not always medically compliant. I was unemployed for many years. I had always been a success and now I was not. My self-esteem evaporated. I was ashamed and embarrassed. I was scared. I was convinced that I was a disappointment to my family and friends. I felt like a burden - for causing them so much worry. I resisted when my family tried to get me help. They didn't always know how. I knew that they loved me very much, but still, I withdrew and isolated myself.

I would often cry myself to sleep. One of the few things that gave me comfort was my cat who never left my side. At times, I felt my life was over. I experienced suicidal depression. I cycled up many times – leading to five severe manic episodes, three involuntary hospitalizations and an arrest for breaking into a house of worship to pray.

Finally, I resigned myself to my illness. But, I was angry and saddened by the stigma society casts on the mentally ill. I, myself, have been called crazy many times. But, sometimes, the most painful stigma is from our own families even if they don't mean it.

At my lowest point, I finally learned about recovery. In the hospital, I was introduced to peer support. Recognizing my condition and sharing with others could help. I was inspired by the example of others, particularly those in like circumstances, with similar backgrounds who could understand me because they had been there too. I was also inspired by substance use recovery examples, which are so often diminished. A seed of hope was planted.

Recovery started slowly, but it built on itself. I returned to something that had always nurtured me – learning. I learned as much as I could about the peer movement. I became a peer support specialist. I embraced the key principles of psychiatric rehabilitation -hope, self-determination, empowerment, an approach centered on the person (not just the illness) with a focus on strengths and recovery. I recognized that the ultimate goal must be wellness – good physical and mental health.

Most importantly, I realized that this battle was not mine alone to fight. I needed my family and they needed me. To be needed is a powerful thing. I asked them for help.

I took ownership of my illness. I did everything I could. I stopped crying and started fighting. I found a wonderful new psychiatrist. He made me believe in a life beyond stability. He cared about my wellness, my dreams and goals. He didn't keep me sedated. Dr. Goldberg and I don't always agree, but he's usually right. I am medically compliant. I'm on lithium, latuda, lamictal, seroquel, and vyvanse. I wish I didn't have to, but I have no choice. My doctor and the right medications saved my life. Therapy helps too. I see a psychologist who is kind and supportive and have seen a family therapist who is caring and helped us when times were hardest. But, the most important therapy has come from my family and friends who know me better than anyone ever will.

Medical treatment and therapy was just the beginning. I had to take better care of myself. I have a healthier lifestyle. I hit the gym four times a week. My diet could be better. Even still, I lost over 60 pounds. I watch for my triggers. I practice coping skills. I feel re-connected to this world. I was able to believe in God again. I still count on my pets – my cat Dude and now a dog – Max - for emotional support. I am engaged with my community. I talk about my condition. I listen to my family. When they tell me I'm not well, I don't push them away. I wish I had accepted their help sooner. I apologized for the hurtful things I said and did while I was ill. I received compassion. I came out to my friends. My closest friends treated me as if I had never been ill at all. I was touched. I was afraid that they might feel sorry for me. We don't talk a lot about my illness, but I love it when they check in on me. It tells me that they care. I was terrified that other friends might reject me. Most were very supportive, and our friendships grew stronger. I felt wanted. I made new friends with those who also have mental illness. They accepted me. I could finally be myself.

I found the courage and strength to believe a normal life was possible for me – a family, a career, happiness. I realized that too many people like me continue to suffer in silence. I wanted to fight for social justice – to combat stigma. I wanted to be an advocate, to help more people like me reach recovery. And, I had to get back to work to be fulfilled. I was afraid and insecure, but I chose to take a calculated risk. With my spouse Izzy's help, I built our online community for people affected by mental illness, substance use or stressful life events. It is a place to not be alone, to share our experiences and inspire and encourage each other to achieve recovery and wellness. It is a challenging project, but I have a wonderful team and mission behind me. I also need your help to make my dream come true, to help as many people as possible, who understand our pain and suffering as only we can.

I have put my full self into this community - my strengths, my struggles, my vulnerabilities, and my passion.

It took me a really long time to get here, but I am now optimistic about life. I will never be my former self, but I am better and stronger to have endured and overcome. My only regret is that I did not get help sooner. I hope you will. But still, I know that I am not cured. There will always be challenges and setbacks, but we can overcome these. Mental illness took me to my greatest depths, but it also showed me the power and resilience of the human spirit. Ultimately it was the unending love of family - Izzy, my mom and dad that pulled me through. With the love of those we love there is nothing we can't overcome.

The battle against mental illness must be won, but we need each other. Ours is a community of great courage and strength.

On Our YouTube Channel: https://bit.ly/39vA5JU

3
Video Script: Talking About Mental Illness
Katherine Ponte

Hello, my name is Katherine. I have bipolar disorder, but I wasn't always talking about it.

My diagnosis was a shock. Everything changed. I was bipolar. I couldn't accept it, yet I couldn't escape it. I just wanted to be normal. I desperately wanted people to treat me as they always had, to be themselves around me. I didn't want everything in my life to change. People only seemed to care about my bipolar disorder. I didn't want to talk about it. If someone forced me, I'd get angry. How could talking about this thing that I hated make me feel any better? What would I say?

I was overwhelmed by stigma. I wondered what everybody else was thinking. I was afraid that I might be rejected. To avoid that conversation, I withdrew. I was trying to protect myself against stigma. Most of my friends respected my wishes to be left alone, but I wish that they had not. I lost a lot of good friends to my mental illness. I still miss them.

A few good friends – Rui, Fabiola, Nuno, Irene, and Tamara, but especially my husband, Izzy and my parents refused to go away no matter how hard I pushed them away. They never stopped reaching out to me, they never gave up. They made me feel loved and needed. They made me feel like the most important things about me had not changed, they made me feel like myself.

We did not talk a lot about my mental illness, but they noticed when I was not well. They asked me about it. They encouraged me get help, but most importantly they gave me the love and support that I needed to take it on. They kept pulling me out of isolation. They showed me that I would not lose everything to mental illness, that they'd always be there for me, no matter how bad things got.

So I felt more at ease opening up. As we all got more comfortable talking about mental illness, we grew even closer together. We realized that we were still the same people.

And we don't always have to talk about mental illness, it's most important to talk about us.

On Our YouTube Channel: https://bit.ly/39yNDo3

4

Video Script: A Caregiver's Mental Illness Journey
Izzy Gonçalves

Hello, my name is Izzy.

Like many families, we have been dealing with mental illness.

In our case, my wife has bipolar disorder. We have been living through the challenges and more recently the possibilities of her mental illness for well over a decade. Through this journey we have learned some personal lessons about what works and doesn't work when adjusting to mental illness as a family. I am sharing our experience in the hope it is useful to others going through a similar situation.

My wife was first diagnosed almost 20 years ago as a grad student, but the real journey for us started with her first full blown manic episode in 2006.

I came home one humid, thundery summer night to find my apartment entrance blocked from within. Music was blaring inside. I finally got in and found my wife raging about religious conflict. It looked like a storm had blown through our tiny apartment.

She was in danger. I didn't know what to do.

I was forced to call 911. Paramedics arrived with several police officers, standard procedure for a psych call. I thought "is this a medical emergency or an arrest?"

The hospital was cold and sterile. A minimum 72-hour hold turned into several weeks in the psych ward – an involuntary hospitalization.

She hated and blamed me for it, said I overreacted. She didn't accept the diagnosis. Later, when she could no longer deny it, she said that I contributed to her illness.

My shock and confusion turned to anger and resentment. How could she blame me?

Yet, I couldn't help but feel guilty. I didn't know what caused her episode. Maybe it was something I did. In fact, a lot had recently happened that could have triggered it – a combination of family stress, work stress, stressful life events. I just didn't know enough to make the connections. Better awareness might have allowed me to recognize her sleepless nights and feverish writing that led up to the episode as more than a productive spurt.

Could It Happen to Me?

Visiting the psych ward was enlightening and humbling. In many cases, I could see past the effects of stabilizing meds to patients who had lives, in better times, like many of us. It made me think how easily anyone of us could end up here for a "time out" from life – maybe only one traumatic experience away. It normalized mental illness somewhat for me.

Shared Experience

My wife and I both had a lot to learn in the coming years about the illness, ourselves and us to ultimately achieve recovery together. There would be several more manic episodes and two additional hospitalizations over ten years.

For so long, neither of us thought deeply about how the other felt or was impacted by the illness. I never thought she appreciated how hard it was for me to become the caregiver while doing my best to keep up at work and sacrificing other things and relationships in my life.

Stigma made me bottle up details and my emotions from family, friends, and colleagues. I internalized my feelings and isolated myself.

We failed to recognize that we shared many of the same intense feelings but hardly ever felt in it together.

Fear

We were both fearful of a now uncertain future. Would insurance cover all of the astronomical costs? Would she relapse? Could she still pursue her career goals?

Helplessness

We felt helpless. Bipolar was a power bigger than us. We didn't know what we could do to prevent or manage it, other than taking the medications. My wife needed the meds, but they weren't enough to reach recovery.

Trauma

We both suffered trauma. I didn't appreciate how traumatic and belittling her hospital experience was. She only recently recognized how traumatic it was for me to witness and try to tame her manic episodes. Signs of a new episode would trigger fear and uncertainty of a repeat for me. I worried how destructive the next one might be.

Hopelessness

Combined with the sedating medication, depression caused my wife to sleep away most of her days. She was inactive, no longer creative, no longer hopeful. And I was no longer hopeful for her.

Loss

We both experienced a feeling of loss. It's actually called "ambiguous loss". My wife was still here, but she was not the same. We were still together, but this was not the life we had envisioned. Couples therapy could have really helped put things in perspective and understand how the other felt. It would have been helpful to talk to other supporters dealing with the same types of issues as well.

Helicoptering

I scrutinized my wife's behavior. This constant watchful hovering is called "helicoptering". My wife hated being under my constant surveillance.

I focused on preventing the next manic episode. I should have focused at least as much on my wife's depression as her mania.

In fact, she was perhaps in greater danger when depressed than manic. In addition to alerting her doctor to more exuberant behavior, I should have identified when she dipped deeper into depression.

Alienation

I was frustrated that my wife didn't take more ownership of her condition. Her doctor and I communicated directly and pretty much controlled her treatment. That made it worse. We thought we knew what was best for her. And so my wife became less secure in her treatment when she saw her doctor and me teamed up against her.

Communication Issues

In fact, my wife started to hide her symptoms from me for fear that I would raise the alarm with her doctor. I now know that she was terrified of ending up back in the hospital. The fact is that we both had the same top priority – to avoid a relapse and involuntary hospitalization for her.

Our communication issues prevented us from working together for this goal. We didn't know how to talk or listen to each other for the longest time.

Ownership

After many years, my wife took a stand, a risk for the prospect of a fuller life.

As she started to find strength and hope from peer support, she wanted to take more control over her treatment. She changed doctors and forced me to adjust my role in her care. I was furious since I also saw signs of a brewing episode. Luckily, her new doctor jumped right into action, and it worked out.

Reconciliation

Her new psychiatrist also advised that we see a couples therapist. He also supplemented her care with a therapist. These additional resources helped open up the channels of communication between us. And we finally recognized that our goals were in fact the same.

Integrated care

With this realization, my wife, her doctors, and I started working together to achieve recovery. We respect each other's roles and motivations and have agreed to certain rules to keep us in recovery.

For example, my wife acknowledges that I am good at detecting her early warning signs. I can share these concerns with her doctor, but she needs to be included in the communication. This type of collaborative care planning would have been a great tool for us to use all along.

We now are better partners in treatment and in life. We do more things together and don't make bipolar the center of attention. We go to the gym together, walk our dog, and eat dinner together as much as possible. We enjoy time in the country. And we also avoid her triggers.

We can both have more control over the condition, reducing fear and helplessness.

Self-care

I also focused on my own care. I suffered from depression and anxiety through the years. My wife finally appreciated the impact her mental illness had on me. She suggested that I start seeing a therapist, which I did.

She also encouraged me to take better care of myself, like seeing a trainer, which I do.

These activities and genuine improvement in my wife's condition have helped. I drew boundaries between her needs and my interests and time. I felt freer to start reconnecting with old friends and exploring new activities. Pursuing these interests made me more engaged, connected, and happy.

I now realize that to be the best caregiver you need to take care of yourself too. Caregivers often sacrifice their own health and emotional needs for the wellbeing of their loved one.

A better life

We reached a better place together which reconciled our former hopes and dreams with the realities of my wife's condition. The ambiguous loss was in fact not a real loss. We didn't lose our former life together. It is just a different life now, and potentially a more fulfilling one.

We gained insights from our experience living with mental illness that should allow us to help others in similar circumstances.

Peer support

That's why my wife built ForLikeMinds, with my support - to make it easier for families affected by mental illness to connect and communicate with each other.

We knew from our experience that it was important to make this a peer support community for people with conditions as well as their supporters.

There is no need for families to face the challenges of mental illness alone. Countless other families can help with peer support, resources, and insights.

The path to recovery can be very challenging for those with conditions and their supporters. But working together it can be a clearer and smoother journey.

I understand the challenges that many of you face. I know from personal experience that it can get better. It did for us, I hope it can for you too and that sharing our story might help.

On Our YouTube Channel: https://bit.ly/2Y2XAEV

5
Bipolar Thriving
Bipolar Recovery Coaching

I created Bipolar Thriving to help other people impacted by bipolar access the benefits of peer support. Peer support restored my hope, which led me to recovery. My goal is for Bipolar Thriving to help others reach recovery as well.

Benefits of Peer Support

It can be useful for people living with bipolar and their families to receive guidance from peers who have been through similar experiences.

We can help families address the challenges and improve relationships. We have first-hand knowledge and experience managing the many issues posed by mental illness.

Our Bipolar Mental Recovery Coaches can help with:

- Fostering and sustaining hope
- Regaining self-respect and self-esteem
- Moving past shame and stigma
- Overcoming withdrawal and isolation
- Countering reluctance to seek help
- Understanding and accepting a diagnosis
- Understanding and seeking treatment
- Knowing what questions to ask your doctor
- Addressing treatment non-compliance
- Talking about difficult topics
- Working as a family unit
- Building and managing personal relationships
- Dealing with relapses and hospitalizations
- Developing and practicing self-care skills
- Transitioning back to work or school
- Achieving and maintaining wellness

We have Lived Experience Expertise in Bipolar I and II, Psychosis,

Depression and Major Depressive Disorder.

The insights of Mental Illness Recovery Coaches may be an excellent complement therapy or other treatments by incorporating mentorship into the recovery process.

Bipolar Recovery Coaches can offer:

- Non-clinical support services to an individual living with mental illness, caregiver, and/or groups that align with SAMSHA's 10 Guiding Principles of Recovery: https://adobe.ly/3cUb2ku

- Personalized, peer-to-peer relationships that support development and use of skills to manage crises and achieve recovery, wellness, and life goals. Their lived experience can help other individuals living with mental illness, caregivers, families, and families-of-choice reach recovery;

- Help initiating treatment and achieving and sustaining recovery. Serve as a role model for recovery by inspiring hope, building confidence, self-efficacy, empowerment, and engagement;

- Help addressing multiple life domains, including physical health, mental health, social health, spiritual health, financial health, and daily living to maximize potential areas for positive change;

- Their lived experience can offer differentiated and unique insights into situations such as suicidal ideation and psychosis;

- Sharing experiences with relapses and hospitalizations and rehospitalizations, which may help reduce relapses and rehospitalizations and / prevent and manage a crisis;

- Personal knowledge to help an individual living with mental illness and/or a caregiver access and navigate reputable resources and support services that can help achieve their goals, including:
  - o the mental health care system
  - o non-profits
  - o online sources of information
  - o education, employment, and social activities

- Extensive experience addressing the challenges of living with mental illness including reaching and staying in recovery;

- Help caregivers better understand the experiences of an individual living with mental illness, enhance their relationship, and support that individual;

- Help an individual living with mental illness and/or a caregiver develop strategies to better communicate with each other and/or friends and family or family-of-choice;

- Help develop and improve working relationships with health care providers, including encouraging the use of shared decision-making;

- Help adopt and use person-centered, recovery-oriented practices in interactions to enhance the provision of services and support;

- Extensive experience living, communicating, and working with their own families and friends to reach recovery;

- Insights from working with other people impacted by mental illness;

- Facilitate mental illness rights and systems advocacy by an individual living with mental illness and/or a caregiver;

- Understand and maintain the privacy and confidentiality of an individual living with mental illness and/or a caregiver;

- Work founded on the key principles of respect, shared responsibility, and mutual agreement;

- An excellent complement to the work of psychiatrists and therapists;

- A potential effective alternative source of support; and

- Convenient remote delivery of insights - including video, telephone, and text.

For more information contact Katherine at
katherine@bipolarthriving.com
BipolarThriving.com

6
Psych Ward Greeting Cards

Inspiration

The Psych Ward can be lonely. We're alone with our own thoughts and reflections — relapses, struggles, disappointments, and hopelessness. I know. I've been there. I suffer from severe bipolar I disorder with psychosis and suicidal depression. A mental health crisis landed me in the psych ward three times. There are rarely get well wishes or flowers for the window ledges. Often, patients have no visitors at all. These were the lows of my struggle with mental illness. I felt locked inside both emotionally and physically.

My mother sends me a stream of get well greeting cards, one a week. They always have a hopeful, encouraging message. They're lovingly and caringly decorated, embellished with stickers, covered with XOXOXOs. They always make me feel better, loved and cared for, remembered, even though I live far from home. I wanted to share these feelings with other patients in psychiatric units when they need it most. I created our Psych Ward Greeting Cards program to do just that.

Program

Psych Ward Greeting Cards makes it easy for empathic and compassionate people to let patients in the psychiatric unit know that people, even strangers, care about them and support them. ForLikeMinds created and manages this program to deliver greeting cards from strangers to patients at participating hospitals. As insignificant as it may seem, sharing a card can have a wonderful impact when a patient is at their lows – offering help, encouragement, and hope. More than 80% of former patients in psychiatric units surveyed said receiving a "get well soon" card would help their recovery. We also share these greeting cards at a highly vulnerable time for patients. Suicide rates after patients are discharged from a psychiatric unit are 100 to 200 times greater than the general population. They need our support at this critical time.

We make it easy to show patients in the psychiatric unit you care.

Donate a card. Send it to us. And we'll deliver it to the psychiatric unit.

Every month we visit the Payne Whitney (Psychiatric) Clinic at New York-Presbyterian Hospital in New York City, one of the country's leading psychiatric units, as well as other participating hospitals. It is an honor and a privilege to support their patients and work with their staff.

If you would like to support patients in the psychiatric unit:

- *Please Donate Cards.* You can send cards with your own message and/or decoration or blank cards. Include an inspirational and hopeful message such as "get well soon", "have hope", "you can recover", or whatever hopeful message you like. Adorn the cards with decorations, stickers, etc. Send the cards to us.

A few considerations:

- We especially welcome cards donated by people affected by mental illness who are many of our contributors.

- Please feel free to send blank cards as well. We helped develop a program for patients in psychiatric units and non-profits to write messages and share cards with each other.

- Please do not include faith-based messages since we currently are unable to control the distribution of cards to individual recipients.

- Please do not include identifying information on the card or card envelopes.

Please partner with us. We would love to partner with you or your organization, including individuals, patients, card artists and designers, card shops, companies, hospitals, non-profits, support groups, schools, clubs, etc. All partners will be featured on our ForLikeMinds Facebook page and in the Our Work section of our program. Please contact us.

Please mail all items to address provided on website.

Testimonial: "Receiving the get well cards from "ForLikeMinds" was a breath of inspiration! Our inpatient peers were very touched, both by the beautiful designs and by the messages of hope and recovery. Knowing that strangers -- some of them in recovery themselves took the time to send these heartfelt messages, gave them a feeling of support and sustenance. In fact, several of our peers decided to make their own cards to contribute to the "ForLikeMinds" program! We look forward to an ongoing connection with this wonderful outreach initiative."

Chaya Weinstein, Occupational Therapist
Payne Whitney Clinic, New York-Presbyterian

PsychWardGreetingCards.com
medium.com/psychwardgreetingcards

Thank you
for allowing us
to be part of
your recovery journey.

Please share your feedback with us at:

hello@forlikeminds.com

Hope is good. Hope works.

Hope captures the power and resilience of the human spirit –

Hope from within, from the love and support of friends and family, from peer support, from recovery examples, from a supportive community.

Hope can and will deliver us from mental illness to a full and meaningful life.

Katherine Ponte, ForLikeMinds

Made in the USA
Coppell, TX
10 April 2021